The Professional's Guide To Teaching Aerobics

Sharon Kay Stoll
University of Idaho

Jennifer Marie Beller
University of Idaho

with Mark S. Moorer

Prentice Hall, Englewood Cliffs, New Jersey 07632

Library of Congress Cataloging-in-Publication Data

Stoll, Sharon Kay.
  The professional's guide to teaching aerobics / Sharon Kay
Stoll, Jennifer Marie Beller.
      p.   cm.
  Includes index.
  ISBN 0–13–161985–3
  ISBN 0–13–161993–4   (pbk.)
  1. Aerobic exercises—Handbooks, manuals, etc.   I. Beller,
Jennifer Marie.   II. Title.
RA781.15.S75 1989
613.7′1—dc19   88-25462
                                                      CIP

Editorial/production supervision and
    interior design: Cyndy Lyle Rymer
Cover design: Diane Saxe
Manufacturing buyer: Peter Havens
Photographer: Mark La Moreaux
Illustrations: Jennifer Beller
Clothes courtesy of Herman Sports and
    The Sport Shack, Moscow, Idaho

© 1989 by Prentice-Hall, Inc.
A Division of Simon & Schuster
Englewood Cliffs, New Jersey 07632

Printed in the United States of America

10 9 8 7 6 5 4 3 2 1

ISBN 0-13-161993-4   PBK.

ISBN 0-13-161985-3

Prentice-Hall International (UK) Limited, *London*
Prentice-Hall of Australia Pty. Limited, *Sydney*
Prentice-Hall Canada Inc., *Toronto*
Prentice-Hall Hispanoamericana, S.A., *Mexico*
Prentice-Hall of India Private Limited, *New Delhi*
Prentice-Hall of Japan, Inc., *Tokyo*
Simon & Schuster Asia Pte. Ltd., *Singapore*
Editora Prentice-Hall do Brasil, Ltda., *Rio de Janeiro*

To Amanda, who made writing this book such a challenge.

Contents

chapter 3
Education in the Sciences: Part Two / 53

chapter 4
Education of Health-Related Fitness in the Aerobic Dance Program / 85

chapter 5
Being Skilled as a Teacher / 103

Preface

This text is developed to help the aerobic dance instructor become a better teacher. Most of the current aerobic texts are anthologies written by numerous exercise professionals. Their contents are general and do not apply specifically to aerobic dance. Therefore the goal of this book is to provide logical, coherent, applicable, and easy-to-read information relevant to the needs of those who teach or administer aerobic dance programs.

This text is based on sound exercise philosophy and specific fitness values. Our aerobic dance instruction policy is founded in the following: 1) commitment to fitness, 2) education about exercise science, 3) skill as a teacher, 4) competence and ability to apply knowledge and skill, and 5) certification by a reputable agency. We believe that these five values are important to be an adequate, effective, and successful aerobic dance instructor.

We would like to acknowledge the contributions made by Natalie Duffy, Mary Mahan, and Debbie Blume Coia in their reviews of the manuscript. We also thank our models, Carol Slavik and John Claycomb, for their time and patience; and Cyndy Rymer, our production editor, for all her time and effort.

chapter

1

A Philosophy for
Teaching Aerobic Dance

INTRODUCTION

Aerobic dance instruction can be exciting and fulfilling. As participants learn about their bodies and the importance of physical fitness, the fitness instructor has immediate intrinsic rewards. The participants see the instructor as someone to emulate: a fit, attractive, fun person. The instructors find themselves held in esteem; they are "important" people.

At the same time, aerobic dance instruction can be professionally frustrating and physically debilitating. Many instructors are not prepared well enough to teach. The American College of Sport Medicine has found that about 90 to 95 percent of all exercise instruction is inadequate. At the same time, many instructors also suffer acute and chronic injuries, and some research suggests that the number may be as many as 75 percent of all instructors. Other studies state that because of frustration and injury, instructors "burn out" quickly and leave the fitness industry, causing a continual turnover rate, resulting in a lack of continuity and expertise.

Because of these problems and inadequacies, new as well as experienced instructors are clambering for more information, and many certifying agencies are attempting to meet the void with clinics, seminars, and tests. The aerobic dance teaching profession has bettered itself, but the certification process has not made instructors foolproof, and they know it. They want information that is logical, coherent, applicable, and easy to read.

We agree. This text is developed to help the aerobic dance instructor become a better teacher. We write this text as a manual with continuity as well as content. Most of the current instructor texts are anthologies, written by numerous exercise professionals. Their content is general and usually does not apply specifically to aerobic dance. We noticed a void of continuity and depth. Therefore, we developed this text based on specificity of knowledge for the aerobic dance instructor. We are experienced teachers in aerobic dance and have based this text on sound exercise philosophy and specific fitness values. Our philosophy about aerobic dance instruction is founded in the following values:

1. Commitment to Fitness,
2. Education about Exercise Science,
3. Skill as a Teacher,
4. Competence and Ability to Apply the Knowledge and Skill, and
5. Certification by a Reputable Agency.

FITNESS

Before we begin, let's discuss exactly what we mean by the term "fitness."

Fitness is often misunderstood and thought to be aerobic conditioning. However, the terms are not synonymous. "Physical fitness" encompasses a variety of meanings ranging from "those characteristics to which a person is able to function efficiently . . ." (AAHPERD, 1977) to "the ability to carry out daily tasks with vigor, without undue fatigue, and with ample energy to enjoy leisure-time pursuits and to meet unforeseen injuries." (President's Council, 1987). To be fit means something different for the Olympic athlete, for professional bowlers, and for the average person on the street. The difference in terminology for fitness stems partly from two varying definitions of fitness:

1. Performance-Related Fitness (PRF) and
2. Health-Related Fitness. (HRF)

PRF

Performance-related fitness is sport-specific fitness. It's the specific fitness that a performer may need for a specific sport activity. As such, performance-related fitness is a measurement of skill, power, endurance, agility, and coordination needed for specific sports.

HRF

In contrast, fitness for aerobic dance instructors and participants should be an acceptable level of the sum total of health-related fitness. HRF is concerned with those aspects of our physical and psychological makeup that afford us some protection against coronary heart disease, problems associated with being overweight, muscle and joint ailments, and physiological complications due to stress. These disabilities and diseases are associated with hypokinetic (less than normal activity) lifestyles. Research tells us that adquate exercise will develop an efficient and effective cardiovascular system, a certain degree of muscular strength and endurance, and ample flexibility. These components of health-related fitness, combined with controlled body weight, good nutrition, and reduced levels of stress, help prevent disabilities and diseases and promote an effective, functional lifestyle. As noted above, the components of HRF are:

1. Cardiovascular efficiency,
2. Muscular strength and endurance,
3. Flexibility,
4. Weight control,
5. Nutrition, and
6. Stress reduction.

COMMITTED TO FITNESS

We believe that for an aerobic dance instructor to be successful, she or he must make a commitment to lifetime fitness. Commitment does not mean obsession. Commitment means being intellectually and emotionally bound to living a wholesome, healthy life. Commitment means believing that exercise is as much a part of life as eating, sleeping, and drinking. Commitment means valuing fitness not just for the changes it makes in physical appearance, but valuing exercise for the changes it makes in mental and spiritual growth. Commitment means believing fitness is fun and fulfilling. Commitment involves a quest for lifetime fitness, practicing daily, and enjoying movement activity. If the instructors can honestly say this is their commitment, they will exude enthusiasm. Fitness does not last just for the length of the program or the sixty minutes that participants attend class. Rather, fitness requires a lifetime commitment.

A Final Note

Once the instructor is committed to health-related fitness, it is time to become educated in the scientific principles and components of fitness. Chapters 2 and 3 will discuss these components of health-related fitness and explain how education based in science is imperative to competent and effective aerobic dance teaching.

chapter

2

Education in
the Sciences

Education about the components and principles of fitness is necessary for effective and competent instruction in aerobic dance. Since fitness is a lifetime commitment, health-related fitness components and principles must be taught in aerobic dance classes.

Before we begin our discussion, let us review the definition of aerobic dance exercise.

AEROBIC DANCE DEFINED

Aerobic dance is vigorous, oxygenated large muscle exercise which stimulates heart and lung activity for a specific period of time to bring about beneficial changes in the cardiovascular system. The main objective of dance aerobics, like any other form of aerobics, is to increase the maximum amount of oxygen that the body can process in a given amount of time. The aerobic effect depends on the body's ability to (a) rapidly breathe large amounts of air, (b) forcefully deliver large volumes of blood, and (c) effectively deliver oxygen to all parts of the body. In simplest terms, the aerobic effect is large muscle activity that brings about a reduction in resting heart rate. Aerobic conditioning is synonymous with the first component of HRF: cardiovascular efficiency.

CARDIOVASCULAR EFFICIENCY

Cardiovascular efficiency, like aerobic dance, is defined as exercise using groups of large muscles to do repetitious tasks for more than two minutes. Certain physiological facts are helpful in understanding the effects of exercise on the chief organ of the cardiovascular system: the heart.

THE HEART

The heart, or cardiac muscle, weighs less than a pound and is generally about the size of a fist. The human heart has four chambers (see Figure 2-1). The two upper chambers, where the veins empty, are called the *atrias*. The two lower chambers, where the blood leaves the heart, are called *ventricles*. The muscle walls of the atrias are thin because, aided by gravity, they only have to pump blood into the ventricles. In contrast, the ventricles pump blood throughout the body. This increased pumping requires a larger force, hence larger muscle.

Blood circulates through the body. It is pumped to the lungs, where it is oxygenated. The oxygenated blood is then pumped back to the heart and then to the body tissue.

At the tissue site, oxygen is exchanged for carbon dioxide. The oxy-

FIGURE 2-1

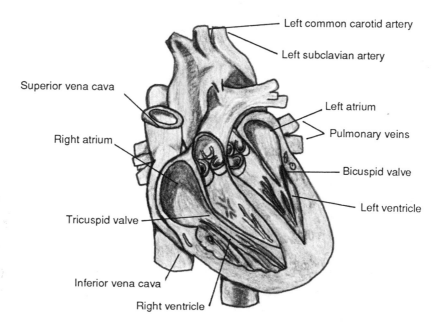

gen in the tissue is used as a source of energy in the cell powerhouse, called *mitochondria*. Blood filled with carbon dioxide molecules is returned to the heart via two large veins, the *superior vena cava*, which brings blood from the head, arms, and shoulders, and the *inferior vena cava*, which drains blood from the body below the heart, into the right atrium. The blood then passes through the tricuspid valve into the right ventricle. From the right ventricle, the blood leaves the heart through the pulmonary artery, which travels to the lungs where carbon dioxide is expelled through respiration. Oxygen is then inhaled. Blood then returns to the heart via two pulmonary veins from each lung to the left atrium. From the left atrium, the blood passes through the bicuspid valve into the left ventricle. From the left ventricle, blood leaves the heart via the aorta to the body and the process repeats.

The amount of blood or volume pumped per one beat is called *stroke volume*. The stronger the heart becomes through aerobic training, using a series of large muscles to initiate training, the greater the stroke volume. Also, the additional work load from aerobic training stimulates the development of coronary arteries, or arterioles, and increases the diameter of the walls of the heart. The result then of aerobic training is a larger heart, with more arteriole supply, which is able to pump more blood efficiently and effectively with less work.

In exercise, the heart's major purpose is to deliver oxygen and nutrients to tissues and to carry waste products away. The greatest amount of blood used during maximal exercise is called *maximum oxygen uptake*, which is an indicator of cardiovascular fitness. It is believed that cardiovascular training can increase about 20 percent of our maximum oxygen uptake, whereas the other 80 percent may be genetically determined.

TRAINING PRINCIPLES

Since the heart is a muscle, a change in its physiological capacity depends on how much work it does. The most effective work load for the heart is to work at a percentage of its maximum capacity *(intensity)* for a specific *duration* and a certain number of times per week *(frequency)*. That means aerobic conditioning is dependent on *intensity*, *duration*, and *frequency* as well as other training principles.

Intensity

In terms of aerobic dance programs, the amount of *intensity* is determined by the age of the participant and his or her level of current fitness. As people age, the normal resting heart rate declines. Therefore, the amount of work load for a younger person is usually much greater than for an older person. Simple formulas such as Karvonen's Maximal Heart Rate Reserve Method or the Maximal Heart Rate Method are used to determine how hard each person should work to achieve an aerobic effect.

Karvonen's Maximal Heart Rate Reserve (HRR) Method

Karvonen developed a method to find the target heart rate to reach during aerobic conditioning. Karvonen determined the heart rate reserve (HRR) as the difference between the resting heart rate (HR_{rest}) and the maximal heart rate (HR_{max}) or

HRR	=	HR_{max}	−	HR_{rest}
(heart rate reserve)		(maximal heart rate)		(resting heart rate)

In order to use this formula, the resting and maximal heart rates must be known.

The resting heart rate can be found by palpating the radial artery (at the wrist), the temporal artery (in front of the ear), the carotid artery (in the neck), or directly at the heart (below the left breast). Be careful to use light pressure, particularly at the carotid artery. Too much pressure will close the artery completely or may cause a reflex that slows the heart rate or triggers cardiac abnormalities. Probably the best time to find the resting heart rate is just before rising in the morning. Try to take the pulse before the alarm startles you.

Count the heart beat or pulse for 15 seconds and multiply that number by 4. The result will be an estimate of resting heart rate for one minute. Do not count the first beat or a counting error will occur. The heart rate is the time between two or more consecutive beats. For an accurate count, start counting from the second beat.

THE MAXIMAL HEART RATE

Outside of an exercise physiology laboratory, determination of maximal heart rate is difficult. However, estimates can be made from the formula:

220 − your age = Maximal Age-Corrected Heart Rate

The number 220 has been estimated as the maximum heart rate for average individuals. To work at this rate stresses the heart beyond its capacity to function effectively and efficiently. Physiological abnormalities, such as arrhythmia, exhaustion, fatigue, fainting, and even death, can occur with too high heart rates. It is not true that exercising at very high levels will bring about fitness faster. Exhaustion and fatigue do not bring about fitness. Fatigue results in diminished work load as the heart works to maintain life functions, such as maintenance of a normal body temperature.

Because heart rates decrease with age, aerobic work load must also decrease with age. To take this into consideration, the above formula is age-corrected to determine maximal heart rate.

220 minus age is equal to maximal heart rate.

220 − _____ = _____ Maximum heart rate.

Because we know that no one should ever work at maximum heart rates or age-corrected maximal heart rates, the question then becomes: how much should we work to bring about cardiovascular or aerobic power? Research tells us that for any muscle to increase in strength it must be worked at 60 to 80 percent of its maximal (or age-corrected maximal rate). Because the heart is a muscle, we can place these percentages (60 to 80 percent) into the Heart Rate Reserve Method. We can then determine heart rate intensity for an aerobic effect.

For example, suppose the resting heart rate was 60 beats per minute, and the maximal heart rate was 200 beats per minute. The heart rate reserve would then be $200 - 60 = 140$ beats per minute. The target heart rate can then be determined as a percentage of the heart rate reserve plus the HR_{rest}. Using the heart rate reserve, a target heart rate of 75 percent of the heart rate reserve would be calculated as found on Table 2-1.

TABLE 2–1 Formula to Calculate Reserve Heart Rate Method.

HRR = 200 − 60 = 140 bpm (beats per minute)
75% THR = (.75 × 140) + 60
165 bpm

For an aerobic effect to occur using the Reserve Heart Rate Method, the exercise must be intensive enough to cause the heart rate to reach 165 beats per minute.

Maximal Heart Rate Method

The target heart rate, to bring about a reduced resting heart rate over a period of time in the maximal heart rate method, is between 60 and 80 percent of its maximum age-corrected rate. These percentages are considered acceptable for untrained populations. A 60 percent of maximal heart rate is known as *Minimal Training Effect* or minimal aerobic effect. This means that the resting heart rate is raised to 60 percent of maximum through large muscle activity for an aerobic effect. The maximum aerobic/training effect is 80 percent of the maximal heart rate. Anything greater for untrained populations may negate the aerobic effect through fatigue and exhaustion.

$$(220 - \text{Age}) \times .60 = \text{Minimal Aerobic Training Effect}$$
$$(220 - \text{Age}) \times .80 = \text{Maximum Aerobic Training Effect}$$
$$(220 - \underline{\quad}) \times .60 = \underline{\quad} \text{ Minimal Aerobic Effect}$$
$$(220 - \underline{\quad}) \times .80 = \underline{\quad} \text{ Maximum Aeobic Effect}$$

Pulse Checks

In order to check whether participants have reached their target heart rates, teach them how to take their pulse during exercise. Although it is difficult to take an accurate pulse during exercise, a 6- or 10-second pulse count immediately following an aerobic dance, while the participants are still walking about, can give a reasonable indication of working heart rate. A 6-second count would be multiplied by 10 and 10-second count by 6 to convert to beats per minute.

Duration

In order to have a consistent aerobic effect, we must perform large muscle activity, raise heart rates to a working effect, and keep it there for at least 20 to 30 minutes. How long the exercise continues depends primarily on the intensity of the exercise and the participant's long-range goals. We do know that beginners should exercise for a minimum of fifteen to 20 minutes. As fitness levels improve, the aerobic session can be increased to 30 minutes. However, as instructors, we must remember that too much too soon will bring about stress-related injuries. After participants have reached 30 minutes of aerobic training, their cardiovascular fitness should be markedly improved. If participants exercise longer than thirty minutes, their goal is not fitness. Instead, their goal is training for some competitive sport event like a marathon.

Frequency

Frequency of aerobic dance sessions should be limited to three times per week. The body needs time to rest and recuperate if fitness is to be developed. The amount of aerobic work results from the intensity of the work, how long it occurs, and how often. This does not, however, mean that if 30 minutes is good, then 90 minutes is better, or that a frequency of seven times a week would be best. There are limits to exercise and its benefits. The result of exceeding these limits is fatigue, exhaustion, and injury.

Besides intensity, duration, and frequency, other principles must be followed if cardiovascular (CV) efficiency is to occur. These principles are

1. Overload,
2. Specificity, and
3. Detraining.

Overload

Stressing an organ or system beyond its accustomed load to bring about a beneficial effect, is called "overloading." Overload stresses the heart, as well as other systems, to accomplish more work compared to previous exercise sessions. For example, during aerobic dance, the participant can lift the legs higher, or swing the arms more. Of course, this overloading has its limits. Once aerobic fitness is developed, maintenance is possible without overload. The overload principle only applies to improving work efficiency.

Specificity

The particular work abilities of selected muscle groups or the exclusive kinds of work to be accomplished involves the principle of specificity. For an aerobic effect to occur, aerobic work must be done; to build muscle strength in the arms, work must be accomplished for that specific muscle group. To train for running a marathon, for example, distance running is required. Flexibility is also specific. To increase the range of motion (ROM) in the shoulder, flexibility work specific to that that joint must be performed. Strength and flexibility are also specific to each muscle or joint. Flexibility in one joint or muscle group does not mean other areas are flexible.

Reversibility

Nonwork reverses the training effect. That is, if exercise is not continued, the aerobic effect will be lost. Complete bedrest can initiate reversibility in a week's time, and cessation of exercise will cause detraining in approximately two weeks. However, if the participant is fit and exercise is ceased for two to three weeks, fitness loss is less and recovery is easier and quicker compared to someone who has never been fit.

Protocol

A training protocol refers to the arrangement of frequency, duration, and intensity during the endurance workout. In other words, each endurance workout is based on the regimen of intensity coupled with duration and frequency. A training protocol, for example, might be an intensity of working at 70 percent of age-corrected maximal training effect for 20–30 minutes per session, three times a week. Training protocols vary as to the specificity of the training; a triathlete has a more intense training protocol—perhaps an intensity of maximal, 5–6 hours per day, 3–5 days per week—than a recreational runner who may have a minimal training intensity—20 minutes per session, three days per week.

EFFECTS OF AEROBIC CONDITIONING

The direct and indirect benefits of aerobic conditioning can markedly improve the quality of life. The direct benefits (Table 2-2) from improved cardiac and respiratory function lead to a decreased change of disease and disability (Table 2-3).

　　Since the heart is a muscle, development of the muscle tissue increases its overall strength. With this improved strength, the concomitant beneficial effects are: improved stroke volume, lowered resting heart rate, increased blood flow to the heart through increase in number of coronary arteries, and a development of respiratory muscles. We have discussed all of these benefits earlier. However, a few others we have not.

TABLE 2–2.   Direct Benefits of Aerobic Conditioning.

1. Lowered Resting Heart Rate
2. Increased Heart Size and Capacity
3. Increased Number of Coronary Arteries
4. Greater Stroke Volume
5. Increased Strength of Respiratory Muscles
6. Increased Overall Bodily Muscle Tone
7. Improved General Circulation
8. Longer Resting Periods between Heart Beats
9. Increased Number of Red Blood Cells and Increased Hemoglobin Levels
10. Decreased Low-Density Lipoproteins, Increased High-Density Lipoproteins
11. Change in Body Compositon
12. Increased Metabolic Rates
13. Increased Caloric Output

TABLE 2-3.   Indirect Benefits of Aerobic Conditoning.

A. A Reduced Chance of
　1. Coronary Disease
　2. Hypertension
　3. Obesity
　4. Lower Back Pain
　5. Arthritis
　6. Osteoporosis
B. A Slowing of Aging Process

Lowered Blood Pressure

During cardiovascular work, lowered blood pressure may occur because more blood is being forcefully pumped through the cardiorespiratory system. It is thought that the force of the blood flow may decrease cholesterol or fatty materials deposited within the arteriole walls. These deposits occur because the connective-tissue layer of a vessel thickens from as early as the age of three. Fatty streaks attach to the arteriole wall and, if not corrected through exercise, will develop to a fibrous plague sometime between the ages of thirty and forty. Another theory is that because of nervous strain or kidney malfunction, resistance is applied to the peripheral arteriole lining. This high blood pressure, called *hypertension*, imposes a chronic, excessive strain on the normal cardiovascular system. At present more than 20 million Americans have high blood pressure and one out of every five persons will have abnormally high blood pressure sometime during his or her life.

Steady exercise such as aerobic dance, jogging, swimming, and bicycling may decrease both systolic (contractile phase of cardiac cycle) and diastolic (relaxation phase) blood pressure. Perhaps a reduction in blood pressure occurs because steady-rate exercise dilates arterioles in the muscles and reduces peripheral resistance to blood flow. However, exactly why blood pressure decreases with endurance exercise is not known. Recent research indicates that blood pressure is reduced through endurance exercise only because the amount of storage fat and intramuscle or tissue fat is reduced. Thus with diminished resistance from the decreased storage fat, blood pressure is lowered. However, other research has found that blood pressure decreases as a result of exercise independent of weight gain. Whatever the reason, exercise directly or indirectly can positively effect blood pressure.

Decreased Low-Density Lipoproteins;
Increased High-Density Lipoproteins

An increased fat (lipid) level in the blood is associated with coronary heart disease. Cholesterol and triglycerides are the two most common lipids. These fats do not circulate freely in the blood, but are carried in a protein called *lipoprotein*. Four different lipoproteins are collectively called *serum cholesterol*: chylomicrons, very low-density lipoproteins, low-density lipoproteins, and high-density lipoproteins. However, not all of these lipoproteins are culprits of heart disease. A high concentration of high-density lipoproteins (HDL), which comprise the smallest portion of lipoproteins, also contains the largest quantity of protein. These high-density lipoproteins may be associated with a lower risk of heart disease. HDL may act as a scavenger of lipids by promoting the movement of cholesterol from the tissues to the liver, where it is excreted with the help of bile. In contrast, low-density lipoproteins (LDL) and very low-density lipoproteins (VLDL) act as transporters of fat throughout the body, including passage through the smooth-muscle walls of the arteries. If too much fat becomes lodged on these walls, the risk of high blood pressure rises as well as the possibility of heart disease. HDL levels are known to increase, however, and LDL levels to decrease, with endurance exercise. Thus, aerobic dance decreases coronary disease risk factors.

Lowered Percent Body Fat, Increased Percent Lean Body Mass

Aerobic dance or any endurance-type activity practiced at an intensity of 60 percent to 80 percent maximum HR three times a week for thirty minutes a day will have an effect on body composition. Specifically, such an exercise regimen will decrease the amount of storage fat in the body and increase lean body muscle mass. Abundant research findings support this concept. For example, a group of athletes was placed on an adjusted diet program and different levels of exercise for ten weeks. Their diets were adjusted to meet the needs of different levels of intense exercise and rest. The results are noted in Table 2-4. The athletes' weight did not change appreciably, but their body compositions did. When training ceased and diet was modified, fat percentages markedly increased. This concept is important for aerobic dance instructors: participants should see a change in body composition with aerobic conditioning.

TABLE 2–4. Adjusted Diet and Exercise Program.

BEGIN ROUTINE TRAINING		INTENSIVE THREE WEEKS	SEVEN WEEKS REST
Weight	116.38	116.82	118.58
Percent Fat	19%	12.9%	17.3%
Calories Consumed	2460	2900	2100

Increased Metabolic Rates Up to 24 Hours/Increased Caloric Output

Research shows that intensive aerobic activity raises metabolic rate. Metabolism is defined as the sum total of processes occurring in a living organism. Because heat is produced by those processes, metabolic rate can be measured by the rate of heat production. In the human body, metabolic rate is measured through the rate of oxygen consumption. The maximum capability to consume oxygen is related to the ability to perform hard work over prolonged periods. A high capacity to consume and utilize oxygen indicates high metabolic function. In order to consume and utilize oxygen and perform work, the body demands more calories for energy. Hence, aerobically fit indviduals and individuals performing aerobic exercise, burn calories at a higher rate.

INDIRECT BENEFITS OF AEROBIC CONDITIONING

Besides the immediate effects to physiological function, aerobic conditioning is known to reduce the chance of disease and disabilities associated with inactivity. Research has found that certain risk factors are associated with coronary-respiratory diseases. Some of these risk factors (such as gender, race, age, and heredity) cannot be alleviated. Males have a higher incidence of coronary-respiratory disease, as do Caucasians, middle-aged individuals, and those people who have a family history of heart or respiratory disease. Obviously, we can do little to change these risk factors. However, other factors such as cigarette smoking, hypertension, elevated serum cholesterol, diet, obesity, physical inactivity, diabetes, and emotional stress, can be altered for the positive through lifestyle modification and commitment to fitness. We will continue to discuss methods to alleviate these risk factors.

Lower Back Pain

Lower back pain is one of the most frequent medical complaints of American adults today. It has been long established that stomach and lower back muscle weakness, combined with inadequate flexibility, are the two main culprits of lower back pain. Exercise can directly affect lower back pain by developing postural muscles (rhomboids, trapezius, sternocleidomastoid) plus stomach (rectus abdominus) and lower back (erector spinae) muscles. Exercise also increases flexibility, as well as indirectly affecting lower back pain.

Arthritis

Millions of Americans suffer arthritis. It is typically a disease of joint stiffness and pain. Numerous forms of arthritis have been found, though generally they all fall within two basic types: rheumatoid arthritis and osteoarthritis. Rheumatoid arthritis generally strikes early and progresses rapidly to bring about deformed joints and general crippling. Aerobic exercise is not recommended, though exercise in water would be highly beneficial. Osteoarthritis appears to be the normal deterioration of joints through constant use and previous injury. Any activity that increases ordinary stress and strain, such as being overweight, poor posture, or working in damp and cold conditions, may bring about osteorarthritis. Specifically designed low-impact aerobic dance, by increasing blood supply to the joint, may be beneficial to osteoarthritis suffers. With increased circulation, tissues become more pliable, which results in an increased range of motion.

Aging

Physiological and performance capabilities generally decline after about age thirty. These rates of decline vary, but are significantly influenced by many factors, including the level of physical activity. Regular physical training appears to enable older persons to retain higher levels of functional capacity, such as flexibility, strength, reaction time, movement time, alertness, and especially CV efficiency. Regardless of age, regular vigorous physical activity produces measurable physiological improvement. The magnitude of these improvements depends on many factors, including initial fitness, age, and type and amount of exercise.

TESTS TO DETERMINE CARDIOVASCULAR EFFICIENCY

For an aerobic effect to occur, we know that groups of large muscles must exercise. But exactly what is large muscle activity?

Large muscle activity refers to vigorous total body execise, incorporating many large muscle groups. Two major goals of aerobic conditioning are (1) to enhance lung and heart circulation capacity and (2) to develop an efficient oxygen consumption system. To accomplish these goals, the mode of exercise for aerobic training must be one that involves the whole body. During total body exercise, a low heart rate and small incremental heart rate increases with more vigorous exercise generally reflects a high level of CV efficiency. This reflects a larger heart stroke volume. Common tests used to measure aerobic capacity are step tests, treadmill graded exercise stress tests, and bicycle ergometer stress tests.

Step Tests

A step test, as does all other aerobic capacity tests, estimates oxygen consumed while performing vigorous work. The participant steps up on a bench or series of steps to a timed cadence, and then returns to the starting position. The step is usually 8 to 16 inches high, involves a cadence of 96 plus or minus with 24 steps up and down per minute, and is three minutes in duration. A pulse count is taken during a thirty-second rest, and scores are compared to given fitness classifications. The Canadian Home Fitness Program offers a good field step test published by Rousseau Publishing Corporation Ltd., 791 St Clair Ave., West, Toronto, Ontario, M6C 1B8. This test is based on three, three-minute steps. The heart rate scales are developed for gender and age. The Home Fit Kit, as it is commonly known, is an excellent step-test measure of aerobic fitness.

Treadmill

Treadmill tests estimate oxygen consumption while the participant walks or runs at varied speeds on level or inclined surfaces. The greater the incline and treadmill speed, the more work that is accomplished. The treadmill is the best means for measuring the cardiovascular system's efficiency. Stress tests, which measure work load and maximum heart work, are usually performed on treadmills in supervised laboratory conditions.

Bicycle Ergometers

Bicycle ergometers estimate oxygen consumption while the participant bicycles at varied speeds and resistance. The bicycle ergometer is not recommended for maximum stress testing since leg muscle conditioning can deter maximum efforts. This test is best suited to individuals whose regular aerobic exercise participation is nonweight bearing, such as swimmers and bicyclists.

Specificity and Aerobic Dance

These examples of aerobic conditioning measurement demonstrate the principle of specificity. Each individual should be tested in a mode similar to their exercise participation. To increase aerobic fitness the same type of work must be performed. Swimming, bicycling, stepping, and treadmill walking and running, are total body activities. The whole body swims, steps, walks, and runs to generate the aerobic effect. Hence, we can say any activity that approximates walking, running, swimming, or stepping are acceptable as aerobic.

Therefore, to define aerobic activities, we know that the exercise must utilize many large muscle groups working together. Examples of total body exercise are those that take the body through space: walking, running, skipping, stepping, hopping, jumping, and swimming. The total body exercise can incorporate any variation of the above and must be continuous for at least 20–30 minutes.

Exercise programs that use isolated muscle groups to fatigue are anaerobic. Anaerobic programs are exercise bouts of short duration. An anaerobic exercise uses alternate energy supplies to release ATP (adenosine triphosphate) to the muscle. Oxygen is not a fuel source.

Therefore, performing isolated, anaerobic exercise, such as leg lifts or fire hydrants, develops specific muscles to sustain particular muscular endurance exercises, but are not aerobic conditioning.

MUSCULAR STRENGTH AND ENDURANCE

Cardiovascular efficiency is incomplete without the second component of health-related fitness: muscular strength and endurance. Strength is defined as the maximum force or tension generated by a muscle or muscles to overcome a resistance. Muscle endurance is the ability to do repetitious contractions of the same muscle groups, such as leg lifts, sit-ups, or push-ups. Often, muscular strength and endurance are confused with muscular power or muscular tone. However, the terms are specific.

Muscular Tone

Muscle tone is the firmness of muscle, the elasticity of muscle tissue in the state of contraction. Muscular strength and endurance both bring about muscle tone. Muscle tone occurs as muscle either increases in size or efficiency. At the same time, storage fat deposits decrease in muscle tissue. The result is firm muscle.

Muscular Power

Muscle power is the ability to exert explosive force. A muscle contains different types of muscle fibers: fast twitch (white) and slow twitch (red). Fast-twitch fibers have energy stores quickly available for muscle work. In contrast, slow-twitch fibers are slower and more efficient in their use of energy. Apparently, the type of fiber, fast or slow, is genetic. Individuals with a predominance of slow twitch can do repetitious muscle tasks easily. These individuals are able to apply muscle contractions over a long period of time.

In contrast, individuals with a predominance of fast-twitch fibers can apply power for short spurts of time. Examples of athletes with a predominance of fast-twitch fibers are track and field sprinters, long jumpers, weight lifters, and so forth. Athletes with a predominance of slow-twitch muscle fibers are endurance runners, long distance swimmers, and so forth.

In aerobic conditioning programs, the development of strength and endurance brings about muscle tone and some muscular power.

Anatomical Structure of Muscle

In order to understand the nature of muscular strength or endurance, some basic anatomic background is helpful. Within the human body, there are three distinct types of muscles: *cardiac* (which we have already discussed), *smooth*, and *striated*.

Smooth muscle tissue, which lines the wall of blood vessels and so forth, is involuntary. Smooth muscle is not affected by exercise.

Striated muscle, or *skeletal muscle,* may be improved through resistance exercise. Striated muscles make up 36 to 40 percent of body weight in women and 44 to 50 percent of body weight in men. There are 434 striated muscles in the body, with 75 pairs working together. They work in teams— as one contracts, another extends. The biceps and triceps represent an example of this antagonism.

Striated muscles are made up of thousands of contractile fibers or cells that are wrapped in connective tissue. Figure 2-2 shows a cross section of a muscle, with a slice removed and magnified. Muscle fibers or cells are grouped together in bundles. The term striated comes from the light (I) and dark (A) bands within one muscle myofibril. Within these bands are the contractile proteins (myosin and actin) that are the basis for muscle contraction.

Contraction is thought to occur as the proteins within one of the bands causes it to slide across another. The sliding decreases the length of

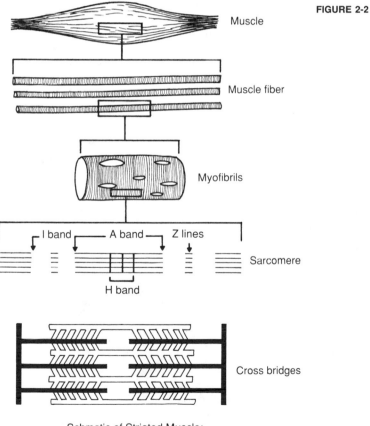

FIGURE 2-2

Muscle

Muscle fiber

Myofibrils

I band — A band — Z lines

H band

Sarcomere

Cross bridges

Schmatic of Striated Muscle:
Showing Z lines, A, H, and I bands

the fiber, causing the muscle to contract or shorten. Striated muscles become stronger by contraction of muscle fibers. Strength increases resulting in hypertrophy (an increase in size of muscle through training); occur either through an increased number and size of the myofibrils per muscle fiber; increased contractile protein within the light and dark bands; increased blood supply; increased amounts and strength of connective, tendon, or ligament tissue; or increased number of fibers.

With hypertrophy strength can also increase. These increases are thought to be the result of greater motor unit recruitment. A motor unit is the functional part of a striated muscle (Figure 2-3). Specifically, a motor unit is a motor neuron and all the muscle fibers that it innovates or fires. Simply put, through a series of electrical-chemical impulses from the central nervous system, a charge is sent to muscle fibers via the muscle nerves. The number of motor units per muscle vary. Muscles of delicate movement like the eye have numerous motor units, whereas muscles of gross movement have fewer motor units. Apparently, motor units also increase in efficiency through use. It is presently thought that females and prepubescent and older males develop strength increases in muscle fiber by increased efficiency of motor unit recruitment; more motor units are called into play during strength training, rather than hypertrophy of muscle tissue.

FIGURE 2-3

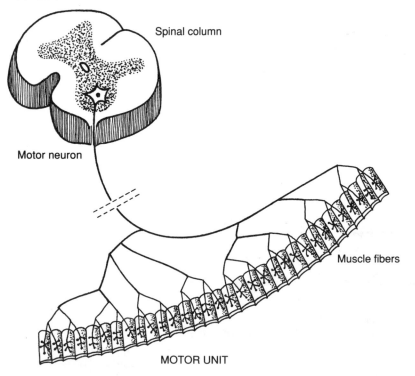

Strength Training and Anaerobic Power

Today, body building and power lifting are often touted as means to fitness. However, most weightlifting programs are inadequate as a means to total health-related fitness because they are not aerobic. In the human body, there are basically three systems whereby energy is made available to muscle cells: two anaerobic systems (phosphagen and lactic acid) and the aerobic system. As mentioned earlier, anaerobic refers to work accomplished without oxygen as a source of energy. In general, the purpose of these systems is to transform chemical energy from food stuffs to mechanical energy. In the human body, mechanical energy comes to fruition in movement. The biochemical process of changing energy from chemical (food stuffs) to mechanical (movement) is indirect.

Energy is first changed to a highly powerful chemical compound called adenosine triphosophate or simply, ATP. ATP is stored in all muscle cells and provides energy for muscles to contract.

The aerobic energy system uses oxygen as a fuel to break down foodstuffs to useable ATP. This breakdown is a complicated process that takes time—at least two minutes to initiate. Hence, physical activities of two minutes or longer use oxygen as the fuel to develop ATP.

In contrast, the anaerobic energy systems, named for their energy sources, use nonoxygenated fuel within the muscle—phosphocreatine and lactic acid—to make ATP. Since these fuels are readily available in muscle, ATP can be instantly utilized. Nature has developed these two anaerobic systems to work hand in hand. As one burns out, or uses up its fuel supply, the other kicks in. However, these fuel supplies are highly limited. Their waste products cause burning muscles after quick, severe bursts of energy. Anaerobic energy is necessary to accomplish short-term activities such as a golf swing, a tennis serve, or a football line play. In fact, any activity of shorter than two minutes' duration is anaerobic. Since most weightlifting protocols are less than two minutes in duration with rest intervals, they are anaerobic and do not develop aerobic conditioning.

To develop muscle strength, endurance, tone, and power, the muscle is dependent on the amount of work accomplished.

Programs to Develop Strength

There are three types of programs to develop muscular endurance and strength:

1. isometric,
2. isotonic, and
3. isokinetic.

Isometric. Isometric (iso – same, metric – length) is a muscle contraction without any lengthening or shortening of the muscle fibers. Figure

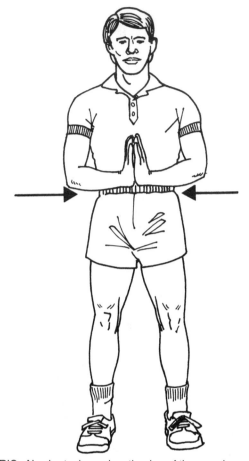

ISOMETRIC: No shortening or lengthening of the muscle as
           it contracts.

FIGURE 2-4

2-4 shows an isometric contraction of the triceps and pectoralis major muscle groups. These muscles are contracting while pushing but are not
lengthening or shortening. Isometrics are fine for rehabilitation programs,
but are not recommended for strength building, since the range of motion
is affected by the type of exercise. Because contractions would have to be
done at every angle in the range of motion, the isometric exercise would
take too long.

    Isotonic.   Isotonic (iso – same, tonic – tension) is a muscle contraction
that lengthens and shortens the muscle. There are two phases of isotonic
contractions: eccentric (lengthens the muscle while in contraction), and

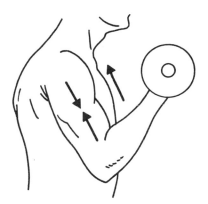

Concentric phase isotonic contraction:
FIGURE 2-5   Biceps shortens as it contracts.

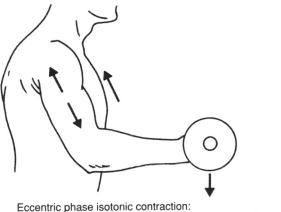

Eccentric phase isotonic contraction:
Biceps lengthens as it contracts.   **FIGURE 2-6**

concentric (shortens the muscle while in contraction). See Figures 2-5 and 2-6 for examples of the two phases of an isotonic contraction. The curl-up phase of a bicep curl is the concentric phase contraction for the triceps (Figure 2-5). It is shortening while it contracts. The curl-down phase is the eccentric phase (Figure 2-6). The bicep is lengthening while it is contracting. Isotonic programs are superior to isometric programs because they develop the full range of motion throughout the contraction stage.

Isokinetic.   Isokinetic (iso – same, kinetic – motion) lengthens and shortens muscle fiber at a constant tension, or resistance, at a dictated speed. Any effort encounters an equal and opposing force—an accommodating resistance imposed by a mechanical device. Isokinetic training makes it possible to activate the largest number of motor units, and to consistently overload muscles, to achieve their maximum force. Isokinetic programs give maximum resistance throughout the range of motion. These programs seem to be superior to isotonic, but because of their high costs, are not acceptable to everyone. Isotonic programs with weights can accomplish the same purpose.

TYPES OF STRENGTH-TRAINING PROTOCOLS

Strength training programs are an excellent way to build strength in specific muscle groups and to develop firmness of muscle. In order to develop strength or endurance, use the principle of overload—that is, to improve the functional capacity of a muscle it must be challenged. Muscles become stronger in response to overload training: working the muscle at 60 percent to 80 percent of its generating capacity is sufficient to produce strength. Four major systems are now used for developing strength and endurance:

1. *Increased resistance through increased weight load* is the most common weight-resistance work. Lifting a certain amount of weight a certain number of times in a certain series of sets to increase the strength or endurance of a specific muscle group.
2. *Increased resistance through repititions of the same weight load* is accomplished by doing a specific exercise a certain number of times, like sit-ups, and each successive session increasing the number of repititions.
3. *Increased resistance through less time to accomplish the same weight load* consists of doing the sit-ups faster and faster each time. Overloading by doing more work in the same amount of time: Time is constant.
4. *Increased resistance through less time between sets* consists of doing repetitions in specific series and reducing the amount of rest between series. For example, doing four sets of 25 curl-ups with a minute rest between set. To increase resistance, keep number of curl-ups the same, sets the same, but decrease time between sets.

Adaptations to Strength Building in Men and Women

Muscular strength is also determined by gender and training. Women are not as strong on an absolute basis since women have only about 36 percent of their total body weight made up of muscle mass and have about four times as much essential body fat, 12.0 percent, as men (gender-specific fat). Men are 44 percent muscle with only 3.0 percent of their bodies essential fat. Regardless of gender, however, muscles generate three to four kilograms of force per square centimeter of muscle cross section. As was stated earlier, women make strength improvements similar to those of men, but without the accompanying muscle hypertrophy, or definition. Lack of hypertrophy in females is probably due to lack of testosterone.

Because of the differences in percentage of muscle to body fat, men are usually stronger than women. But when allowances are made for body size and composition differences caused by gender, strength is about equal, and in some cases women are stronger than men.

A good strength-training or endurance-training program will tone muscle and reduce the amount of body fat for both genders. Strength-training programs (using greater amounts of resistance for fewer repetitions) build muscle quickly. These programs are believed to develop muscle mass, with large bulk and little flexibility, though not necessarily. Flexibility, the range of motion in a joint or series of joints, is lost only when a muscle is not worked throughout its range of motion. Because of the inefficiency of the body's predominate third-class lever system, many individuals who strength-train with heavy loads do not use a full range of motion.

A third-class lever functions through force over a fulcrum to move resistance. An example of a third-class lever is the biceps brachiallis, the elbow joint, and the resistance applied at the hand while lifting weight (Figure 2-7). The fulcrum is the elbow joint, the force arm is the biceps attached at the ulna, and the resistance is the weight of gravity plus any additional weight pulling down on the hand. When the elbow is completely extended and the hand is loaded with a weight, the angle of the forearm (ulna and radius) and upper arm (humerus) muscle is 180 degrees. Since the biceps origin is located in the upper arm, the contraction is at an inefficient position. In contrast, as in Figure 2-7, at an angle of 90 degrees and less this lever is highly efficient, since the force arm is now shorter. We are very strong at 90 degree or less but very inefficient at over 90 degrees. Lifters typically attempt to lift what they can maximally at the more efficient 90 degrees or less angle. The result is cheating in the lift. They will not or cannot lift the load during the inefficient 180 degree angle. As they lift, they fail to work conscientiously (through the full range with a lighter load or with a spotter helping) on increasing or maintaining their flex-

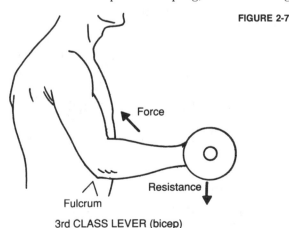

FIGURE 2-7

Force

Resistance

Fulcrum

3rd CLASS LEVER (bicep)

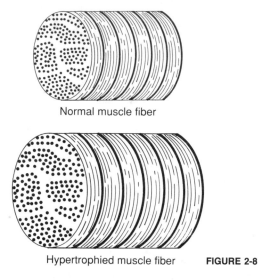

Normal muscle fiber

Hypertrophied muscle fiber   **FIGURE 2-8**

ibility. By violating the principle of work through the full range of motion, they gradually lose flexibility.

Besides loss of flexibility, it is thought that strength training will bring about muscle boundness or bulgy muscles. When muscles become stronger in males, hypertrophy occurs (Figure 2-8). As we discussed earlier, as hypertrophy occurs with weight training, the myofibrils increase in circumference and become thicker. However, a muscle does not increase in length; it can't because adult bones do not increase in length. Consequently, as muscles become thicker, they appear shorter because the muscle cannot increase in length.

In contrast, the same aesthetic effect does not occur in muscular endurance training. As you remember, muscular endurance is the ability of a muscle to do repetitious tasks, and occurs by doing a task over and over again (push-ups or sit-ups, for example). In progressive-resistance programs with added weight, doing frequent repetitions of a biceps curl with a weight is endurance work. Besides increasing the amount of muscle endurance, the muscle becomes toned and appears long and defined. In this case, muscle fibers increase in the length of the muscle in an equal proportion as the muscle hypertrophies.

Both programs (strength training and endurance training) develop hypertrophy, and both develop strength. Strength training develops strength and less endurance, while endurance training develops the muscle's ability to do a lengthy amount of work.

Endurance-Training and Strength-Training Programs

Endurance training can be any type of calisthenic in which a muscle group does the same exercise over and over again. Good aerobic dance choreography develops muscular endurance through most of the body's major muscle groups. Specifically, the choreographed dances should highlight and develop the eight major muscle groups: Shoulders, upper arms, abdomen, buttocks, front of thighs, back of thighs, front of lower leg, and calves. **No other endurance calisthenics are necessary**, except for stomach, lower back, and chest. These three areas are typically difficult to address in aerobic choreography. Their anatomical location is isolated from the groups of large muscles involved in aerobic conditioning such as quadriceps, hamstrings, deltoids, biceps, triceps, trapezius, and so forth. Exercising the abdomen, chest, and buttocks through a full range of motion is better accomplished through isolated endurance training.

Examples of Muscular Endurance Training

We have chosen some examples of exercises that will increase strength and endurance in these specific sites: abdomen (curl-ups), chest, shoulders, and upper arms (push-ups), and lower back (dorsal curls). In each of these exercises, the muscle contraction is done against the resistance of body weight and gravity. Through overload, attempting to do more repetitions in a constant time, muscular strength is improved. By increasing the number of repetitions but keeping weight and time constant, we can develop muscular endurance. We use a 30-second clock for curl-ups and dorsal curls (Increased resistance by increasing repetitions but keeping time constant). Push-ups are *not* performed with a clock (increased resistance by increasing repetitions).

The Curl-up

The sit-up (or curl-up) is performed to a 30-second timed clock. The participant attempts to perform as many sit-ups as possible in the allotted time, and overloads the muscle group by attempting one more on each subsequent trial. The participant lies supine with legs flexed and feet soles flat on the floor, while a partner holds the ankles. The hands are placed across the chest (Figure 2-9). Some participants do not have enough strength to do the curl-up. They often rock and pull their arms forward to accomplish the sit-up. To stop this problem, the arms can be stretched forward beside the thighs (Figure 2-10). The participant keeps the trunk curled with chin on sternum (Figure 2-11). A partner holds the ankles for good leverage and to force muscle action in the lower four inches of the rectus abdominous muscle (Figure 2-12).

Electromyographical studies (electrodes—sensors—placed on muscle to register muscle impulse) show that the sit-up (curl-up) is the best exercise to develop the major longitudinal abdominal muscle: the rectus abdominus. The rectus abdominus inserts at the pubis and orginates at the sternum. Contraction of this muscle flexes the trunk and holds the truck and

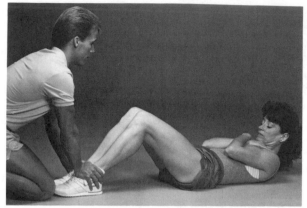

FIGURE 2-9

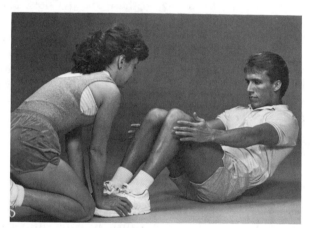

FIGURE 2-10

FIGURE 2-11

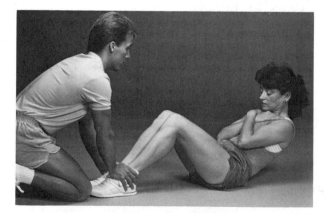

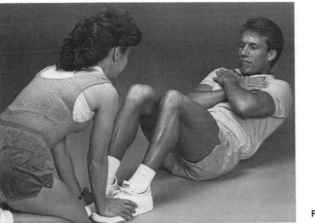

FIGURE 2-12

abdomen securely. The rectus abdominus is often referred to as the girdle muscle because of this support capability.

The lower four inches of the rectus abdominus has higher action potential (muscle work) when feet are stabilized than if feet are not stabilized. Flexing the trunk to 45 degrees and returning to a supine position primarily develops the rectus abdominus. Hence this is the best exercise to develop the rectus abdominus.

If an individual cannot lift the torso to 45 degrees, the partner should reach over, keeping one hand on ankles, and clasp the participant's elbow, pulling them up to the sit-up position (Figure 2-13). A sit-up is an isotonic exercise with concentric (shortening) and eccentric (lengthening) phases. This means that the rectus abdominus contracts while shortening, (the sit-up action), and contracts while lengthening, (the sit-down action). If a participant cannot perform the concentric action (the more difficult of the two), the eccentric phase will develop the rectus abdominus. Hence, by

FIGURE 2-13

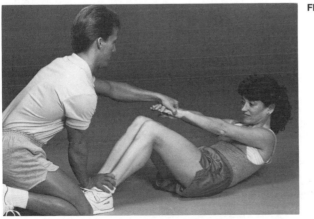

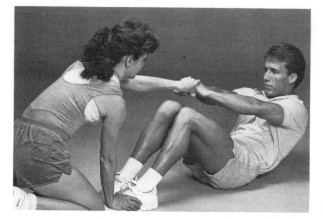

FIGURE 2-14

helping participants through the concentric phase and encouraging them to contract through the eccentric phase, the rectus abdominus becomes stronger (Figure 2-14). In time, participants will be able to perform both phases by themselves.

The Push-up

The push-up, performed from a prone position, develops chest (pectoralis major), upper posterior arms (triceps), and shoulders (rhomboids, deltoids, and trapezius). The hands are palm down under the shoulder. The toes are curled under and grip the floor (Figure 2-15). The push-up is initiated by keeping the body tight and straight. The body is pushed from the floor until the arms are straight (Figure 2-16). The arms then flex at the elbows and slowly lower the body one to two inches from the floor (Figure 2-17). The action is then repeated until the participant cannot perform any more.

Women typically have difficulty with a push-up because of a diminished muscle mass, anatomical design, and little exercise that focuses specifically on the shoulder and upper arm area. During puberty, women's hips widen as the pelvis becomes deeper and wider to prepare for possible pregnancy. The femur rotates outward in the pelvic joint, the acetabulum,

FIGURE 2-15

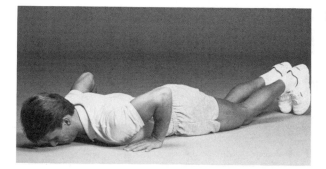

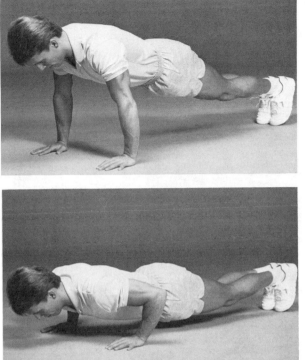

FIGURE 2-16

FIGURE 2-17

as the femur turns obliquely inward. These biomechanical disadvantages combine with 10 percent less muscle mass and 12 to 15 percent more fat to make a lower center of gravity. Also, females typically have narrow shoulders with a wider pelvis which results in the carrying angle of the arm rotated outward. Women must push-up their heaviest body part, the hips, suspended from between the push off points of the hands and feet.

We therefore recommend a four count push-up that accommodates the inefficiency of the female anatomy. The participant assumes a prone position, with palms on floor under shoulders, fingers pointed straight ahead (Figure 2-18). Count 1: push up to a position where arms are

FIGURE 2-18

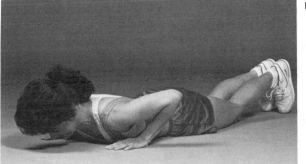

straight, body straight from head to knees, head up, weight supported on hands and knees (Figure 2-19). Count 2: continue to push up to a position where the weight is supported on hands and balls of feet (Figure 2-20). Count 3: lower the body until chest and knees almost touch floor (Figure 2-21). The body is held straight. Count 4, relax the body to the floor. The second push-up continues promptly.

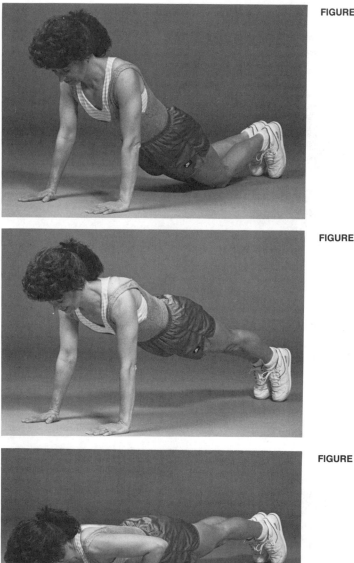

FIGURE 2-19

FIGURE 2-20

FIGURE 2-21

Make sure that count two is a straight body position (women typically will push too high [Figure 2-22]), and that position three is a straight body. Women often sag at the hips (Figure 2-23).

If the participant cannot do a four count push-up, modify the push-up with the help of a partner. The partner lifts at the hip for count 1 (Figure 2-24), follows through count 2 (Figure 2-25), and supports through

FIGURE 2-22

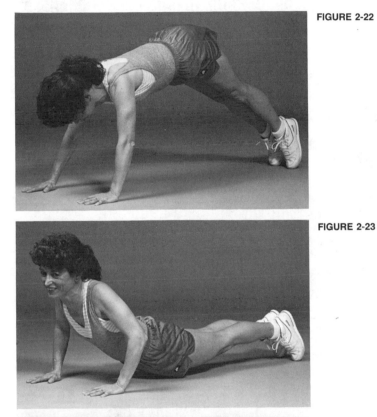

FIGURE 2-23

FIGURE 2-24

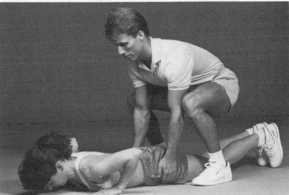

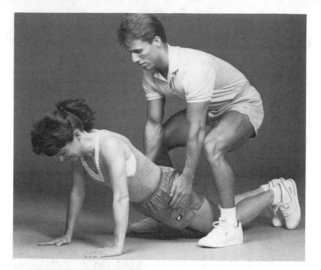

FIGURE 2-25

FIGURE 2-26

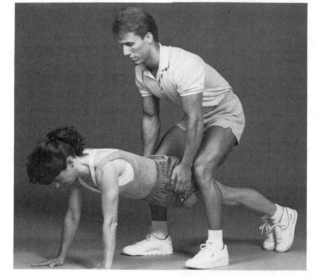

FIGURE 2-27

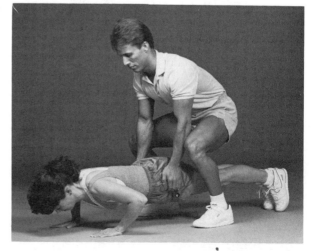

count 3 (Figure 2-26) and lifts at hip to counteract the inefficient mechanical angle (Figure 2-27).

The Dorsal-curl

The dorsal-curl is performed in a supine position facing the floor. The hands are clasped behind the neck (Figure 2-28). The partner sits astride the participant's ankles and presses down on the backs of the thighs to prevent movement. The participant raises head and shoulders from the floor by arching upper back (Figure 2-29). Repeat as often as possible in 30 seconds. The dorsal-curl is not recommended for participants with a history of back pain or injury.

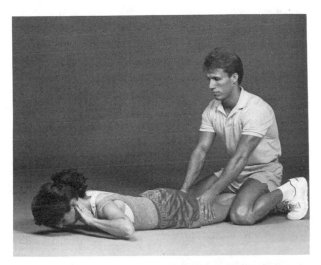

FIGURE 2-28

FIGURE 2-29

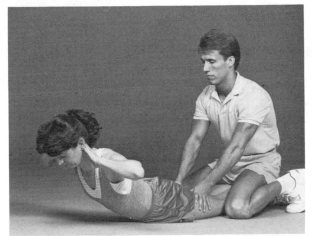

Standards for Curl-ups, Push-ups, and Dorsal-curls

We do not recommend standard tables for endurance training. We believe that the best method to motivate participants is to let them set their own standard. Of course, standards do give participants a goal. However, a better goal would be a percent increase of their beginning level. For example, if a participant scores 15 curl-ups on the first trial, her goal might be a 50 percent increase in 10 weeks, or a total of 23 curl-ups.

How to Develop Muscular Endurance-Training Protocols

As we stated earlier, isolated exercises should only be included in a specific strength-building section. We believe that including such isolated exercises in the choreography compromises the aerobic effect. However, if the instructor believes that additional endurance exercises are necessary, certain questions must be answered:

1. What muscle group is to be developed?
2. What exercises address that group?
3. What progressive resistance system is appropriate?
4. What training protocol should be used?

What Muscle Group.   When the participant chooses the muscle group to be developed, it is important to understand what that muscle group does. If the participant wants to develop shoulders, the instructor must ask specifically which part of the shoulder. Once the specific area is determined, the instructor must educate the participant about how the muscle group functions. Too many times, participants want to develop one muscle group but are exercising a different group. Table 2-5 lists exercises that address each major muscle group of the body.

What Exercise Addresses That Group.   Because of the principle of specificity, choosing the correct endurance exercise is important. The instructor and participant must understand how the muscle group functions and then select the appropriate exercises. See Figures 2-30 and 2-31 and Table 2-5.

We recommend a specific exercise for females to develop the trapeziod muscle. Typically, this muscle is very weak in women. Figures 2-32 and 2-33 show a method to develop strength in the mid-trapeziod region of the upper back. Lie in a prone (on stomach) position. Straighten the left arm perpendicular to the body. Rotate the thumb so it is pointing toward the ceiling and hold (Figure 2-32). Lift the arm straight to the ceiling and hold (Figure 2-33). Properly performed, the arm must be perpendicular to

TABLE 2–5.   Exercises that Address Major Muscle Groups.

EXERCISE	MUSCLE GROUP
Push-ups modified and full	:Triceps brachii, pectoralis major
Hip raising (lie on back, soles of feet on the floor, knees bent)	:Back extensors Gluteus maximus, Gluteus medius
Curl downs	:Rectus Abdominus, Internal and External Obliques
Shoulder shrugs	:Trapezius, Levator Scapulae
Arm curls with palms upward	:Biceps brachii, Anterior Deltoid

Four position leg lifts
  Side Leg lifts
  (hip abduction)
  Inner Thigh Raise
  (hip adduction)
 	
  straight leg raise:
  sitting (hip flexion)
  straight leg raise:
  prone (hip extension)
	
	:Gluteus Medius, Tensor Fasciae Latae
	
	:Gracilis, Adductor Longus, Adductor Brevis, Adductor Magnus
	
	:Rectus Femoris, iliopsoas, iliacus
	
	:Gluteus Maximus,
	Hamstring Group
	(Semimembranosus, Biceps Femoris, Semitendinosis)

Back hyperextension	:Back Extensors, Latissimus Dorsi, Trapezius
Push with palms together	:Biceps brachii and Pectoralis Major
Pull with fingers interlaced	:Triceps brachii, Rhomboids, Posterior Deltoid, Biceps brachii
Neck Isometrics	:Trapezius, Platysma, :sternocleidomastoids
Half squats	:Quadricep Group (Rectus Femoris, Vastus lateralis, Vastus Medialis, Vastus Intermedius), Tibialis Anterior
Calf raises (Toe raises)	:Gastrocnemius, soleus
Full leg and buttock tightening	:Gluteus Maximus, Gluteus Medius, Gluteus Minimus, Hamstring Group, Quadricep Group, Tibialis Anterior, Gastrocnemius, Soleus
Mad Cat (on hands and knees, arch back and hold)	:Rectus Abdominus

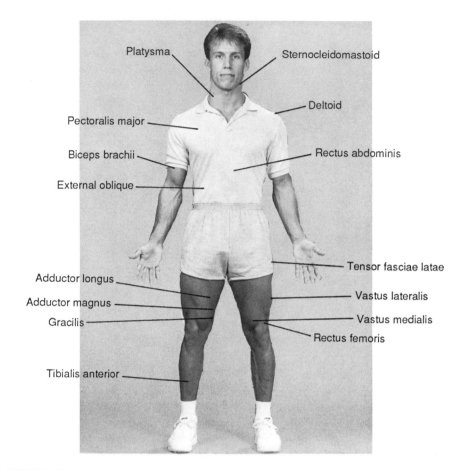

FIGURE 2-30

the body and the thumb pointed skyward. Many women will be unable to lift the arm in this position. Encourage them to work on this both in and out of class. Shortly they will feel strength improvement. Repeat with both arms.

Figure 2-34 shows a method to increase neck and upper back strength. Stand or sit with the head over the shoulders and shoulders back. Place the right index finger on the chin. Gently contract the neck and shoulder muscles toward the back; hold, relax, and repeat. This will increase strength for upright posture and reduce neck and shoulder fatigue from sitting at a desk.

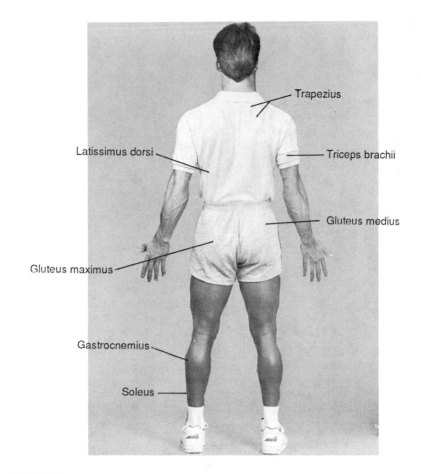

Trapezius

Latissimus dorsi

Triceps brachii

Gluteus medius

Gluteus maximus

Gastrocnemius

Soleus

FIGURE 2-31

FIGURE 2-32

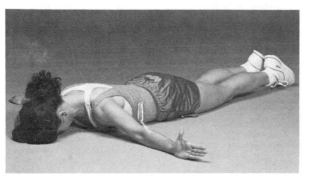

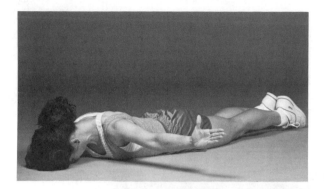

FIGURE 2-33

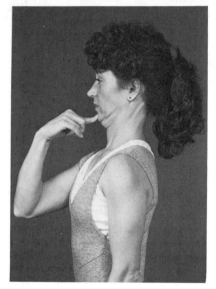

FIGURE 2-34

What Progressive Resistance Is Appropriate.   Endurance training is limited to the progressive resistance systems in which an exercise is done for numerous repetitions, done against a clock, or done with rest between sessions. However, the instructor must also remember that in order for muscle endurance to increase, the exercise must be practiced at least twice weekly and preferably three times per week. These factors bring about a two-fold problem: the chance of stress injury and spending too much time on one muscle group. The instructor must weigh the benefits against the detriments of numerous isolated endurance calisthenics.

What Training Protocol Is Appropriate.   In weight training, the protocol is the amount of weight lifted (intensity), the repetitions of each lift (duration), the sets of the repetitions (duration), and the number of training bouts per week (frequency). For endurance training, the frequency would be the aerobic dance sessions, the intensity and duration would be the length of time devoted to each muscle group.

STRENGTH-BUILDING EXERCISES

In order to develop strength in a muscle, we recommend using increased resistance by increasing the number of repetitions of an exercise but keeping the time of the exercise bout constant, or increase resistance by decreasing the amount of time between sets of the exercise bout. Obviously, this is the same protocol as in endurance training.

As with increasing endurance, the participant and instructor must decide which muscle group to work, the appropriate exercise and protocol. The protocol must be limited within the aerobic dance session so that all the components of fitness are addressed.

Use of Hand Weights

Many instructors and participants feel that by adding hand-held or leg weights their heart rates will increase, causing cardiovascular improvement. This is especially true of participants in low impact aerobic classes. However, current research does not show a significant increase in heart rates or cardiovascular efficiency due to the addition of hand-held weights. Rather, the repetitive stress and addition of hand-held or leg weights causes a significant increase in microtrauma to the involved joints. This microtrauma may result in either curtailment or limitation of participation. The addition of 1-to five-pound weights to the wrist, hand, or leg significantly increases shoulder, knee, hip, or back stress.

Torque is the movement of a segment about an axis. Torque is produced when the muscles of the shoulder and arm contract to raise the arms overhead. Physical laws state that the farther the force arm is from the rotary point the greater the force produced at the pivot point. In addition, the forces at the shoulder joint substantially increase with the arms perpendicular to the body, as in arm circle movements. Arms held overhead or down to the side produce less force at the shoulder joint because forces fall close to or within the line of gravity.

Consequently, with the addition of hand-held weights the forces are appreciably increased at the joint. Microtrauma then occurs to the soft tissues surrounding the joint. Under normal circumstances the body is able to contain the inflammation process. However, the addition of weights causes such a great increase that the body is unable to overcome the stress, and injury occurs.

To increase muscular strength or tone requires many repetitions of the same movement. This repetitious movement causes significant joint stress, violates the repetitive movement principle discussed earlier, and is insignificant in producing strength or heart rate increases.

Therefore, we recommend the avoidance of hand-held, wrist, or leg weights during aerobic exercise. Additional strength increases are met through a vigorous strength-training program separate from the aerobic program.

Muscle Soreness from Strength and Endurance Training

Generally, muscle soreness occurs to everyone who is involved in strength- and endurance-training programs. It is almost impossible to avoid some discomfort and soreness due to the physiological process of increasing muscle strength.

Muscle soreness is usually described as two different kinds: acute and delayed.

Acute Muscle Soreness

Acute muscle soreness occurs while or immediately following exercising. Acute soreness is really only a nuisance during exercise because it disappears after cessation of the exercise bout. It is thought that acute soreness is caused by a lack of adequate blood flow (ischemia). Apparently in acute muscle soreness, pain occurs as blood flow is occluded as muscle contracts. Waste products cannot be removed, hence pain occurs and continues until the contraction ceases or is reduced.

Delayed Muscle Soreness

Delayed muscle soreness is what most of us suffer in strength and endurance training. It occurs after the exercise bout. Unfortunately, unlike acute muscle soreness, delayed muscle soreness does not cease when exercise stops. The soreness usually is greatest two days after the exercise bout. The cause for delayed muscle soreness is unknown, but three theories are currently available:

1. The torn tissue theory espouses that the muscle fibers are actually torn as the strength or endurance work occurs. As the protein in the contractile muscle tissue stimulates the sliding bands, a tearing occurs within the fiber.
2. The spasm theory suggests that when ischema occurs, a spasm results as the nerve endings within muscle fiber are pinched.
3. The connective tissue theory states that the tendons and connective tissue within the muscle are injured during contraction.

Whatever the physiological reason for delayed muscle soreness, two preventive measures can reduce the problem. (1) Stretching after exercise appears to help reduce delayed soreness. Apparently, stretching helps limit the build-up of fluids and lactic acid within the muscle fibers. Blood is prevented from pooling; hence, less fluid build-up. (2) A slow warm-up to full exercise also decreases delayed muscle soreness probably because the muscle becomes warmer as more blood flows to the fibers. The more blood during exercise, the less pain later.

Developing muscular endurance and strength should not be a painful endeavor. Some discomfort may occur but not to the degree that participants refuse to return to class. The best strength and endurance program for the aerobic dance participant is one especially suited to his or her needs. The wise instructor evaluates the current strength and endurance level of each participant and then prescribes an exercise protocol.

FLEXIBILITY

The third health-related fitness component is flexibility. Flexibility is defined as the range of motion (ROM) in a joint or a series of joints. Flexibility is specific to each joint and not equally distributed throughout the body. Range of motion in most joints is limited by connective tissue such as: tendons, ligaments, aponeuroses (fibrous attachment from muscle to bone), and muscle fascial sheaths; bone structure, contact of tissue masses with adjacent areas, and clothing restrictions.

The connective tissues tensile strength tends to increase with exercise, thus promoting a greater range of motion. Consequently, the more variety in exercise activities, the greater the overall range of motion in each joint. In addition, flexibility varies with age. Older persons are less flexible compared to younger persons because muscles become less elastic and connective tissue more tense with age. The aging process can be impeded with consistent, varied exercise activity and participation in cardiovascular and strength programs. Three factors are related to flexibility:

1. *Elasticity*,
2. *Plasticity*, and
3. the *Stretch Reflex*.

Elasticity

Elasticity is the muscle's ability to stretch beyond a normal resting length and return without injury. However, the elastic component of the muscle has a point of no return; if stretched too far, the muscle can herniate or rupture. This occurs when a tendon, which attaches muscle to bone, tears from an insertion, or when the muscle itself tears from too great a strain.

Prevention of a rupture or tear is easy. Warm up completely before exercising. Perform flexibility work; stretch all the muscle groups. When participating in strength building or toning, work through an entire range of motion. Warm down well. Following a good exercise regimen and developing muscles equally will preclude a severe muscle injury.

Plasticity

Plasticity involves the phase where the tissue remains stretched. The permanence of the stretch length depends upon how much plasticity occurs. The plasticity phase is directed towards increasing the viscosity of connective tissue fluid.

The contribution of elasticity and plasticity to flexibility is dependent upon three variables: (1) the amplitude of the force, (2) the duration of force, and (3) the tissue temperature. Generally, moderate forces, for longer durations, with elevated tissue temperatures will increase connective tissue elongation.

Stretch Reflex

The muscle and elastic tissue have a reflexive protective device known as a *stretch reflex*. This electrical, mechanical, and chemical system collects information about the state of muscle stretch. Afferent muscle fibers (muscle fibers within the muscle that serve only as sensors) act as muscle sensors and send information to the central nervous system (CNS). If the muscle is stretched too far and potential for injury is imminent, the afferent muscle fibers warn the CNS, and information is sent back to the muscle via the efferent muscle fibers to reduce the stretch. Unfortunately, this system is not instantaneous, requires a few milliseconds, and cannot override violent, dynamic actions (see Figure 2-35). The figure is of an arm holding a book. Let us assume that the book was just placed in the hand, the force is then pushing downward. In order to keep the book from dropping to the floor, the biceps contract. The figure shows how afferent information (from the biceps) travel to the central nervous system via the spinal column. Efferent information is then sent to the biceps' motor neurons. This whole process takes time. Applied to aerobic dance, we can then infer that bouncing in a stretch to increase flexibility is too quick for the system to warn about potential danger. Hence, injury occurs through minute tears to the muscle itself or to the elastic tissue. Muscle tears are nasty and may be accompanied by hematomas, swelling, and pain. However, because muscles have ample blood supply injury recovery time is approximately six weeks. In

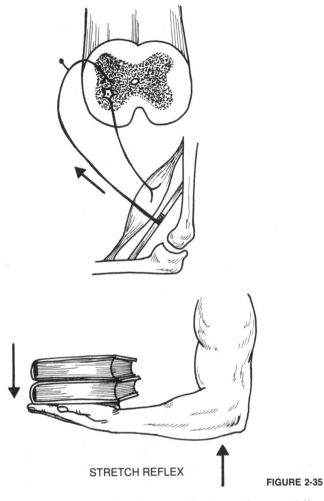

STRETCH REFLEX

FIGURE 2-35

contrast, connective tissue such as tendons and ligaments have low blood supplies and may require a longer recovery period.

Either of these injuries is possible in aerobic dance. The important point to remember is to avoid overloading the stretch reflex. Use a stretching protocol that is static and completely warms the muscle groups involved in the activity.

Through the principle of overload, flexibility in any joint can improve. Remember this means stressing an organ or system beyond the load normally accustomed, thereby causing a beneficial effect. To increase flexibility for aerobic dance participants, gently stress the muscles a little more each time. The overload principle requires time, and flexibility is limited by individual anatomical structure. However, this does not mean that flexibility should be ignored; nor does it mean gradual, almost imperceptible, increases in flexibility are not worth the effort. The total range of motion required to perform any given skill is as great as the sum of flexibility in all joints involved.

Flexibility Exercises

Below are examples of flexibility exercises for the major joints and muscle groups.

Shoulders and Arms.   Figures 2-36 and 2-37 show a method to stretch the posterior shoulder and middle upper back muscles. In Figure 2-36 the left arm is bent, with the right arm holding the left elbow. Using the right arm, gently pull the left arm over the right shoulder. In Figure 2-37, the right arm is held straight. Use the left arm to pull the right arm across the body. The stretch should be felt on the posterior surface of the left shoulder. Stretch both shoulders.

Figure 2-38 shows a simple stretch for the triceps and top of shoulders. With the arms overhead, hold the elbow of the right arm with the left hand. Gently pull the right elbow behind the back. Repeat with both arms.

To stretch the anterior portion of the shoulders, arms, and chest, refer to Figure 2-39. Place the palms of the hands facing each other (the

FIGURE 2-36

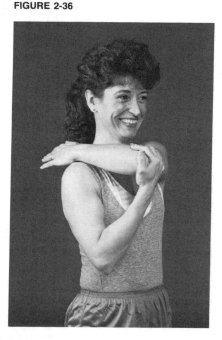

FIGURE 2-37

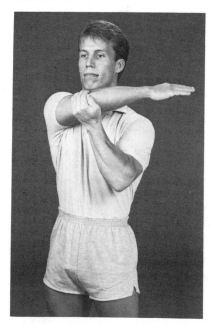

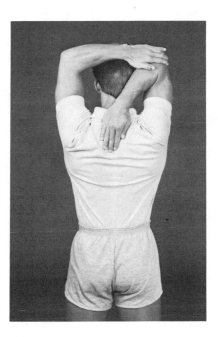

FIGURE 2-38

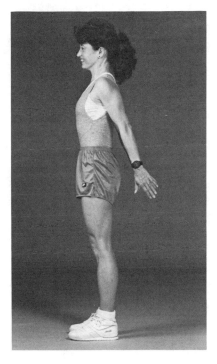

FIGURE 2-39

fingers can be interlaced). Keep the arms straight, chest held upright, and lift the arms up behind the back. For a variation, with the arms straight roll the elbows inward.

Lower Back. Stretching the lower back involves the hip extensors (the hamstrings) and hip flexors (rectus femoris and iliosoas) as well. These muscles attach on both the legs and lower back regions. Figure 2-40 shows a

FIGURE 2-40

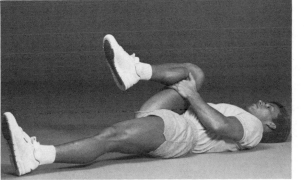

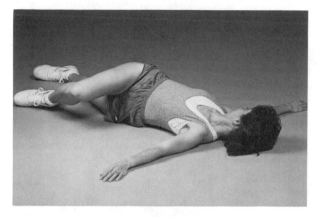

FIGURE 2-41

method for stretching the erector spinae muscles in the back, and the hamstring muscles in the upper leg. Lie flat and push the pelvis to the floor. Use both hands to hold under the bent right knee. Gently pull the right knee to the right shoulder while keeping the pelvis and right shoulder flat on the floor. The pelvis must remain flat on the floor for a proper stretch to occur. Repeat the motion with both legs.

Figure 2-41 demonstrates a stretch for the low back rotary muscles and side of hip. The right knee is bent at 90 degrees and placed across the straight left leg. The arms are perpendicular to the body with the head facing the right arm. Gently push the right knee towards the floor. Ensure that the shoulders are flat on the floor. Repeat with both sides.

Hamstring, Quadriceps, and Lower Leg. The hamstring muscles (upper posterior thigh) are easily stretched using the methods in Figures 2-42 and 2-43. Figure 2-42 shows the hurdlers stretch. The right leg is held straight with the toe pointed to the ceiling. The left leg is bent with the foot placed

FIGURE 2-42

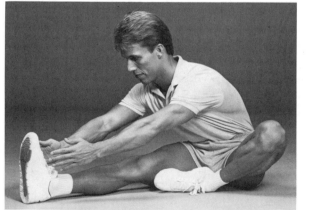

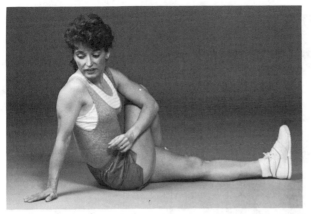

FIGURE 2-43

next to the right knee. Keep the head upright and gently stretch both arms toward the right ankle. Repeat on both sides.

Figure 2-43 shows a modified hurdlers stretch. This will stretch the upper hamstring, upper and lower back, side of hip, and rib cage. Keep the left leg straight, bend the right knee, and place over the left knee. Bend the left elbow and place it to the outside of the right knee or thigh. With the right arm resting behind, slowly turn the head to look over the right shoulder, while rotating the upper body toward the right arm and hand. Repeat with both legs.

Figure 2-44 shows an *improper* method to perform the hurdlers stretch. The right foot is turned outward, the head is thrust forward, and the right knee is bent with the foot away from the body. With the knee in this position, extreme pressure is placed on the left joint capsule, thus creating undue ligament stress.

The quadriceps muscles (front of upper leg) can be stretched by following the method in Figure 2-45. Assume a starter's position. The right knee is bent at 45 degrees and the hands and arms used for balance. The

FIGURE 2-44

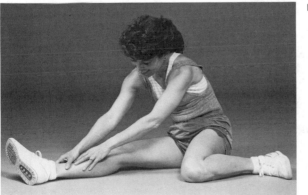

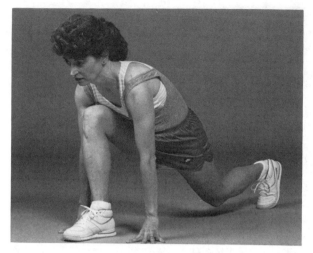

FIGURE 2-45

left leg is stretched behind the body. Slowly lower the hip toward the floor. The straighter the left leg is kept the greater the rectus femoris and iliosoas (hip flexors) stretch. As the left leg is bent the remainder quadriceps muscles receive a greater stretch. Repeat with both legs.

Figure 2-46 demonstrates a method to stretch the soleus muscle (one of the two muscles that insert to form the common achilles tendon). The right knee is bent with the left leg behind the body, knee slightly bent. The heel should remain flat on the floor with the toe pointed straight ahead.

FIGURE 2-46

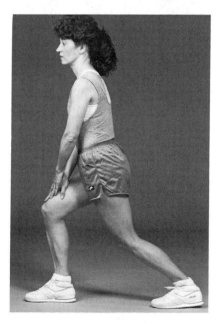

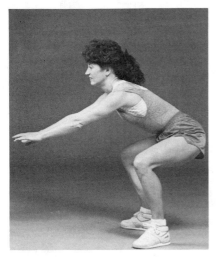

FIGURE 2-47

Gently lower the body until the right knee is approximately 45 degrees. Remember to keep the left heel flat on the floor. Repeat with both legs.

To stretch the gastrocnemius muscle perform the same stretch as in Figure 2-46, only this time keep the left leg straight. Repeat with both legs.

Of the many stretching-flexibility exercises, most are beneficial, but a few are not: standing toe touches with a locked-knee position and feet together put too much strain on the knees, hips, and hamstrings. The "plow position" with feet over head and touching the floor, places too much stress on the neck for most persons. Deep knee bends are unacceptable because of hyperflexion of knees. If pliés are used, make sure that the body is held in alignment and not with buttocks back (Figure 2-47). Any stretching exercise that requires bounding movements should be avoided. Flexibility work may feel tight, but it should not hurt. Keep in mind that flexibility is one of the six components of fitness and that it is as important as the other five.

A Final Note

Aerobic dance is an oxygenated system of many large muscle exercises that stimulate heart and lung activity for a period of time to bring about beneficial changes in the cardiovascular system. The main objective of aerobics is to increase the maximum amount of oxygen that the body can process in a given amount of time.

Strength is defined as the force applied to a resistance. Muscular endurance is the ability of a muscle to apply repeated contractions.

Flexibility is the range of motion in a joint or series of joints.

The five important *training principles* to follow in developing aerobic power, strength, and flexibility are: intensity, duration, frequency, overload, specificity, and reversibility.

As applied to a program of aerobic dance, the instructor must remember that cardiovascular efficiency warrants a program of many large muscle groups which take the body through space. Aerobic dance exercise protocols should follow the same procedures as any other aerobic exercise program.

chapter

3

Education in the Sciences: Part Two

WEIGHT CONTROL

Weight control and nutrition are the fourth and fifth components of health-related fitness to be included under the education value of our aerobic dance program. Because of our affluent lifestyles, weight control is the most difficult fitness component to attain. Four out of five Americans are overweight. Of that number, 50 million men and 60 million women, between the ages of 18 and 79, arc obese.

For our purposes, the term overweight refers to heaviness above the norm or exceeding maximum weight listed by gender, height, and frame size in a standard weight table, such as the Metropolitan Life Insurance Desirable Weight Charts. Obesity is being overfat and having excessive storage fat. Unfortunately, both terms are relative since weight charts are typically in error.

The Metropolitan Life Insurance Company of New York developed tables of desirable weights for men and women in 1960 (see Table 3-1). The data was formulated from averaged weights of thousands of individuals. The problem with such a descriptive method is that the averages are of thc population in general. The tables do not reflect average weights for fit populations. In 1983, the Metropolitan Company revised their weight charts from information gathered in 1979.

TABLE 3–1   Desired Weights for Men and Women, 25 Years of Age.

HEIGHT FEET INCHES	SMALL FRAME	MEDIUM FRAME	LARGE FRAME
MEN			
5 2	112-120	118-129	126-141
5 3	115-123	121-133	129-144
5 4	118-126	124-136	132-148
5 5	121-129	127-139	135-152
5 6	124-133	130-143	138-156
5 7	128-133	134-147	142-161
5 8	132-141	138-152	147-166
5 9	136-145	142-156	151-170
5 10	140-150	146-160	155-174
5 11	144-154	150-165	159-179
6 0	148-158	154-170	164-184
6 1	152-162	158-175	168-189
6 2	156-167	162-180	173-194

HEIGHT FEET INCHES	SMALL FRAME	MEDIUM FRAME	LARGE FRAME
WOMEN			
5 0	96-104	101-113	109-125
5 1	99-107	104-116	112-128
5 2	102-110	107-119	115-131
5 3	105-113	110-122	118-134
5 4	108-116	113-126	121-138
5 5	111-119	116-130	125-142
5 6	114-123	120-135	129-146
5 7	118-127	124-139	133-150
5 8	122-131	128-143	137-154
5 9	126-135	132-147	141-158
5 10	130-140	136-151	145-163
5 11	134-144	140-155	149-168
6 0	138-148	144-159	153-173

(From Metropolitan Life Insurance Company of New York, 1960)

These tables showed a marked increase in the average desirable weight. The scientific community has clearly stated that such increase in the supposed desirable weight charts are deleterious to achieving optimal weights. Americans are already too fat and too unfit.

Also, such weight charts do not account for fat gain accompanying the aging process. An unusual phenomenon occurs as we age. Approximately 3 to 7 pounds of lean body mass disappears every ten years after the age of 30. Typically, this lean body loss is replaced by storage fat. Exercise may slow the process, but cannot completely prevent it.

To place this in perspective with the Metropolitan Weight Charts, let us assume that a 25-year-old, 5-feet 5-inch female weighed 120 pounds and was 20 percent body fat. We monitored her weight and fat percentage for 20 years. She exercised aerobically three times a week and led a fairly active life. At age 45, she still weighs 120 pounds but is now 28 percent body fat. The difference in percent body fat is acceptable with the phenomenon of degeneration of lean body mass. If she had gained twenty pounds in that 20 years, as many adults do, the increased weight would have been totally storage fat and her percent body fat would be markedly higher.

Some researchers believe that this loss of lean body mass loss should be compensated by an accompanying weight loss. Others believe that the increased storage fat, provided no additional weight is gained, helps decrease potential injury and disease. Whatever, all researchers agree that adults should avoid excess weight gain.

Because weight charts are inaccurate or unacceptable as a predictor of desirable weight, scientists state that ideal weight should only be determined in relation to age, gender, lean body mass, and acceptable percentage of storage fat. The number of pounds we weigh should not be the final factor in deciding if we need to lose or gain weight. Rather, we should determine percent of body fat, then compare that percentage with acceptable levels for our gender and age. Acceptable percentages of body fat are relative by age:

Adults:	20-29 years	30-39 years	40-49 years	50-59 years
Men:	>15%	15-18%	18-20%	24-26%
Women:	22-25%	26-29%	28-30%	30-33%

Gender Differences

Certain physiological and anatomical differences preclude a greater percentage of body fat for women compared to men. Because of physiological needs for childbearing, women possess four times as much essential fat as men.

Body fat is divided into two different types: essential fat and storage fat. Essential fat extends through the marrow in the bones, as well as in the heart, lungs, liver, spleen, kidneys, intestines, muscles, and lipid-rich tissues of the central nervous system. This fat is essential for normal physiological functions. In the female, essential fat also includes sex-specific fat stored primarily in the mammary glands and pelvic region. Storage fat, the second major accumulation of fat, occurs in adipose tissue. These nutritional reserves include the fatty tissues that protect the various internal organs from trauma, as well as the large subcutaneous fat volume deposited beneath the skin's surface.

Proportional distribution of storage fat is similar in both females and males.

Athletic Amenorrhea, Anorexia Nervosa, Bulimia, and Other Eating Disorders

If females become too thin, certain dangerous physiological changes occur. A female who drops below 12 to 13 percent body fat may no longer have a normal menstrual cycle—the effect is called *amenorrhea.* Amenorrhea may occur because the loss of storage fat and perhaps essential fat places the body in jeopardy if pregnancy would occur. Research does show that females who regain a normal weight experience a return of menses and can bear children. The long-term effect of amenorrhea is unknown, though it does have such effects as decreased levels of estrogen plus early osteoporosis. Loss of estrogen seems to precipitate chronic soft tissue injuries, stress fractures, early osteoporosis with bone loss, dowager hump syndrome, weakened bone structure, and so forth.

Athletic Amenorrhea. Amenorrhea is also a problem for athletic women. Known as *athletic amenorrhea,* this type of amenorrhea is a constant problem for world-class athletes and dancers. However, according to current research the cause is not decreased body fat. Rather, excessive weight bearing activities such as running and dancing lower estrogen levels, and this possibly causes the amenorrhea. This incurred amenorrhea is a direct link to osteoporosis and bone mass degeneration. A female athlete may be amenorrheic and realize the danger, but find herself in a push-pull cycle. She must train, but the training causes more bone loss. The harder she trains, the more stress she suffers. To compound the problem, many of these athletes eat poorly and have inadequate sleeping habits. Combined with the work load, the result is either amenorrhea or olimenarchy (irregularity) of menstrual cycles.

Anorexia Nervosa. *Anorexia nervosa* is self-starvation. While anorexia was first recognized about 100 years ago, the death of singer Karen Carpenter heightened public awareness of it. The typical anorexic tends to be a young female, a high achiever in school, and often a perfectionist. Usually she comes from a well-educated family. She has an overriding concern for weight control and body image. She will do almost anything to lose weight: abstain from food, use laxatives or amphetamines, and exercise obsessively and compulsively. She typically has a weight loss of at least 25 percent of her original body weight, but a weight loss of 15 percent with a downward spiral may also indicate anorexia.

An anorexic will deny that she needs help. In fact, she will emphatically state that she is too fat and can identify areas of fat on her body, such as the fat fold between the thumb and index finger. She will insist that her bony body is normal and even attractive. She will resist all offers of help and will become resentful and hostile if she is urged to eat. She often wears sizes too large or hides behind heavy sweatsuits.

Physiologically, amenorrhea will set in as her estrogen level drops. This will lead to the inability of bones to absorb calcium with varying degrees of osteoporosis resulting. Lanugo (soft, baby hair over the body) is common. She will have a lower resting pulse, lower core temperature, and her extremities will tend to be cold and even cyanotic (blue-gray in color) due to reduced oxygen to tissues.

Psychologically, she is often introverted and withdrawn, alone, and lonely. She can only be helped through professional counseling. The reasons for the weight loss are psychological, not physiological.

Bulimia. Bulimia is a seemingly uncontrollable food craving that leads to frequent binging and purging. A bulimic again is usually female between the ages of 12 and 30. She may eat two to three times the amount of food in an average meal. She usually swallows high calorie foods such as doughnuts, ice cream, and candy. She then purges herself by vomiting, laxative abuse (sometimes using between 40 and 80 doses or more per day), diuretics, and enemas. Her binging and purging periods may occur monthly, weekly, or daily, depending on the stress in her life. Her binge leads to guilt and fear that she will gain weight, which in turn leads her to purge. After the purge, she is exhausted, but peaceful, and again in control.

She keeps her vomiting secret, but telltale signs of scarred fingers (pushing them down her throat and cutting them on her teeth) and broken blood vessels around the eyes will give her away. Her cheeks may also become puffy from swollen salivary glands.

Physiologically, the extreme diuretic or laxative abuse upsets the electrolyte balance, chemicals that maintain constant heart beats, and she becomes a prime target for heart failure. She may also suffer a ruptured stomach or esophagus. The stomach acid will in time erode her teeth enamel. A continuation of the problem may lead to her death through heart failure or malnutrition.

She will often seek help, not because of the binging but because she can no longer afford her habit. A binge is the cyclic period when she eats and purges. A binge may last as long as a day or as short as a few minutes. Her consumption of 3,500 to 40,000 calories per binge and her ingestion of diuretics and laxatives is beyond her economic means.

Psychologically, she may be more social than the anorexic but usually she is severely depressed and even suicidal. She too needs counseling immediately.

The aerobic dance instructor has a good chance of encountering individuals with eating disorders. However, the instructor is not a professional counselor and should not pose as one. If the instructor suspects that a participant has a disorder, the first step is to help these individuals seek competent help. Some hints to direct these individuals toward help are

1. Do not confront the participant, rather be understanding. Avoid discussing how thin, pale, sick they may look. Instead, show interest in a supportive way. At some time, they may be willing to risk confiding in the instructor if they do not feel threatened.
2. If trust is established, try to get the participant to seek help. You might make contact with the counseling service and accompany the participant to the first session.
3. Bring speakers to the studio to discuss eating disorders in an intimate friendly atmosphere. This may set the stage to help the participant get help.

Help is available in most communities through counseling sevices. If more information or referral is needed, contact: Anorexia Nervosa and Related Eating Disorders, Inc., P.O. Box 5102, Eugene, Oregon 97405, (503) 344-1144 or National Association of Anorexia Nervosa and Associated Disorders, Box 271, Highland Park, IL 60035, (312) 831-3438.

Other Eating Disorders.   Eating disorders also include individuals who eat too much. In fact, the majority of eating problems in this country is related to overeating. As aerobic instructors, our task is to help our participants find the best and most nutritious way to lose weight.

Obesity

We believe that obese populations should not be enrolled in an aerobic dance class. If obese participants enroll, they should be directed to another aerobic program, preferably a nonweight bearing activity like swimming.

Unfortunately, a great many persons in this country cannot control their weight. About 110 million people are classified as obese or grossly overweight (above 30 to 35 percent body fat.)

Obesity occurs in two different ways: Adult onset and childhood onset. Adult onset, *creeping obesity*, results from gaining a few pounds every year for a number of years. With a two-pound increase every year, the change in weight does not seem that significant, but in ten to twenty years the effects are obvious. Physiologically, gross obesity is known as fat-cell hypertrophy. As more fat is deposited, the available fat cells become even larger.

Childhood onset, or *hyperplasia*, is the laying down of excess fat cells during childhood growing spurts. Childhood onset can begin as early as the last trimester of pregnancy, or through age one, when excessive fat cells are developed. These cells will not decrease with weight loss. Once they are laid down, they are in the system forever. A fat cell biopsy conducted on a grossly obese man (328 pounds) to count the number of fat cells in his body revealed 75 million, with a fat cell size of 0.9 micograms. After a period of starvation, the man weighed 165 pounds, and the fat cell size had decreased to 0.2 micrograms, but the cell number was still 75 million. The fat-cell size decreases, but once developed, cells never decrease in number, and they fill with fat easily. The obese person, therefore, is never really cured of his or her obesity (in terms of the number of fat cells present). Research reveals that generally it is possible to decrease body weight in grossly obese persons but it is nearly impossible to maintain that decrease over a number of years. The explanations given for this problem are the irreducible number of fat cells and a host of behavioral problems. In fact, because of the difficulties of treating severe obesity, the focus of research has shifted to a search for factors that cause obesity, rather than finding a solution for the existing problem.

Causes of obesity range from environmental influences to possible prenatal and neonatal (first month after birth) feeding to dietary fat ingestion. The abundance of food is an environmental influence. Our society has too much food with a high caloric value. A dinner with a super burger, large fries, a soft drink, and a cherry pie contains 1261 calories. Low levels of physical activity are another environmental factor. Stress is still another every-day factor. Persons under stress often reduce it by eating more food. Many of us eat when we are anxious or bored. Often, persons who eat more become further stressed by the gain in weight, which causes them to eat even more.

Neonatal feeding and ingestion of dietary fat are other causes of obesity. The long-term effects of the neonatal feeding are associated with a permanently fixed appetite and body weight at higher-than-normal or lower-than-normal levels. Apparently, the mechanism regulating voluntary food intake is fixed to some extent by the amount of food consumed in the first months of life. Babies that are fed high-fat, high-caloric diets have higher fat percentages and more constant appetites than babies who are fed low-fat, low-caloric diets. A fat-rich diet stimulates the appetite. High-fat foods make us eat more.

Implications of Obesity

The implications of obesity and of being overweight are: (a) a higher susceptibility to disease. The overweight have a greater incidence of gall bladder disease, gout, diabetes, hypertension, and arteriosclerosis. (b) A higher recovery risk in surgery, pregnancy, and fractures. Because they have irregular menses, obese women often do not know that they are pregnant; and they recover slowly after giving birth, and often are troubled by other complications. (c) Greater difficulties in respiratory and pulmonary function; a higher incidence of respiratory and pulmonary disease, which often results in functional disability and a decreased life span. (d) Withdrawal from society because of the psychological implications within a thinner society.

Family eating patterns influence the chance of obesity. A greater incidence of obesity occurs when parents are also obese: in 40 percent of all cases both parents are also obese; about 80 percent have one parent who is obese, and less than 8 or 9 percent have parents of normal weight.

The only solution to obesity is the development of a sensible diet and the examination of patterns for children from the third trimester of pregnancy to adulthood.

Ideal Body Weight

Even though anorexia nervosa, bulimia, and obesity are common problems, most participants will not have these concerns. Most will believe they are overweight, and they may be. However, before we recommend weight loss programs, we must first determine their ideal body weights.

The ideal percent body fat depends on several variables: percent lean body weight (muscle, bone, organs, skin, and so forth), percent essential body fat (gender-specific fat, insulation), and storage fat.

Many methods are available to ascertain percent body fat. Laboratory methods range from examination of cadavers to underwater weighing. Field methods use girth measurements or skin folds. Both laboratory and field methods must be done by qualified professionals. Attempting to take skin folds without practice under qualified supervision will result in large error factors, and we do not recommend it.

We also do not recommend programs using electrical impedance to find percent body fat. This system is based on the theory that lean body mass has more water than fat. By measuring the electrolyte fluid balance within muscle, the instrument can estimate the percent body fat. However, the instrumentation is inaccurate, either because individuals are not hydrated enough or the machine is in error. Typically, electrical impedance indicates a greater percent body fat than is actually the case.

The best method to measure body fat is in the laboratory using hydrostatic weighing. This system is based on Archimedes' principle that a mass displaces its own volume in water. Through use of a mathematical fomula, the laboratory technicians can calculate the percent lean body mass and storage fat. Obviously, this method must be performed by qualified personnel.

Another technique which can be used by nonprofessionals employs only a tape measure. For men, measure the circumference of the waist, exactly at the level of the belly button, with the tape held firm in the horizontal position, do not allow the tape to slope upward or downward. Use a ruler to line up the waist circumference or girth with the body weight. The relative body fat is the point where the straight edge crosses the percent fat line. In Table 3-2, a waist girth of 34 and a body weight of 170 gives a fat percent of about 17 to 18 percent.

For women, the circumference is measured at the hip's widest point and the subsequent measurement is used with height to estimate body fat, see Table 3-3.

TABLE 3-2   Estimation of Relative Fat in Men from Body Weight and Abdominal Circumference.

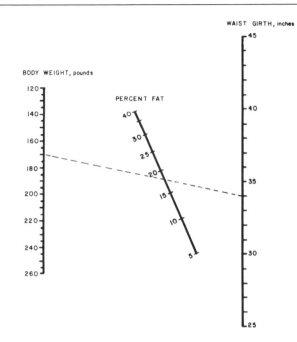

Source: Wilmore, Jack. *Sensible Fitness.* Leisure Press: Champaign, Illinois: 1986, p. 30.

Once percent body fat and lean body mass is estimated, calculation of ideal weight can begin. Table 3-4 is a method to estimate ideal weight. Before calculating, discuss with the participants what percent body fat they would like to be. If their ideal weight is not appropriate, either too high or too low, the instructor would be wise to counsel them on the values of good nutrition and acceptable fat percent levels. We also must remember that no one should begin a weight loss program without counsel from their physician. The estimation table gives percentages and pounds that the participant can understand and set a goal toward attaining.

How to Lose Weight

If the participant is considering a weight loss program, it is time to discuss the elements of weight loss. A successful weight loss is based on five essential principles: exercise, exercise routines, diet, nutrition, and food and the pattern of its consumption.

Exercise. Exercise is the most important of the five principles for weight reduction and control. Research reveals that weight cannot be nutritionally controlled without exercise. Unfortunately, most diet programs

TABLE 3-3 Estimation of Relative Fat in Women from Height and Hip Circumference.

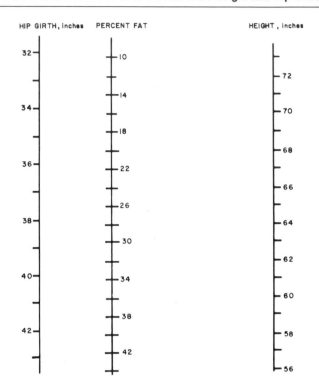

Source: Wilmore, Jack. *Sensible Fitness*. Leisure Press: Champaign, Illinois: 1986, p. 30.

TABLE 3-4 Estimation of Ideal Weight.

1. Name: _____ Gender _____ Age _____

2. Current Weight _____

3. Percent Body Fat _____

Determining Selected Target Weight

4. Current fat weight _____
   [Current body weight (#2.) × Percent body fat (#3.)]

5. Current lean body weight _____
   [Current body weight (#2.) − Current fat weight (#4.)

6. Desired percent body fat _____

7. Estimated target weight _____
   [Current lean body weight (#5.) − Desired percent body fat (#6.)
   1.00

8. Estimated pounds to gain or lose _____
   [Current weight (#2.) − Estimated target weight (#7.)]

rely only on reduction of calories to control weight. It is true that a reduction of calories is the key to weight loss, but it is essential that the proper minerals, nutrients, and vitamins are not sacrificed in the weight loss program.

The best means to reduce weight is to eat properly and increase the caloric output through exercise. Research has established that a nutritional diet balanced with sufficient exercise is the key to a fit, trim body. For example, a research program on the effects of diet and exercise placed three groups on a regimen of 500 fewer calories per day. The first group ate 500 fewer calories per day. The second group restricted its diet by 250 calories per day, but increased its exercise to burn 250 more calories per day. The third group simply increased its exercise to burn 500 more calories per day. At the end of the study all three groups had a weight loss of 12 pounds. The difference in fat loss and increase in lean-body mass, however, was interesting (Table 3-5). Group 1 had a fat loss of 9.3 percent, with a decrease of lean-body mass (muscle and connective tissue) of 2.4 pounds. Group 2 had a fat loss of 12.6 percent, but increased lean-body mass of 1.1 pounds. Group 3 (exercise only) loss 13.1 percent body fat and increased lean body mass to 1.98 pounds. Obviously, the third group became leanest, thinnest, and trimmest, though Group 1 and 2 lost the same amount of weight. The conclusion: the only way to become fit and trim is through strenuous exercise.

Exercise Routines.   Exercise is individual and the energy spent is dependent on several variables: caloric cost, age, size, and activity level. The aging phenomenon also affects our metabolic rate. As we age, we burn calories less efficiently. Some research maintains that this phenomenon is due to a less active lifestyle rather than age.

We also know that larger people burn more calories per minute than smaller people. The greater mass needs more calories to maintain metabolic functioning.

To lose a pound of fat, the caloric cost must be 3,500 calories. That is to say, the amount of energy output must be increased by 3,500 calories or the food intake must be decreased by the same amount. Research has recently shown that this formula is not necessarily true for some obese persons. However, it is true for most individuals.

TABLE 3-5

	GROUP 1	GROUP 2	GROUP 3
	DIET	DIET AND EXERCISE	EXERCISE
Fat loss	9.3%	12.6%	13.1%
Lean-body mass	−2.4 lbs	+1.1 lbs	+1.98 lbs

Men burn more calories a minute per pound than women. Men have more muscle mass and less percent fat. The larger percent muscle mass means a higher metabolic rate. Men, therefore, are more efficient and burn calories faster than women.

Exercise routines are individual; each person has unique physiological functions. A fitness program must be developed around these differences and take them into account. Some women, because they have a lower center of gravity with greater fat pads at the hips, do not like to run. As stated earlier, this lowered center occurs for females at puberty. The pelvis widens; the femur rotates outward at the acetabulum; fat is deposited at the hip and thighs. This increased gender-specific fat is important for child bearing. However, the increased fat plus the widened hips and rotated femur cause inefficiency in running. Such women can choose alternative exercise like swimming, walking, or dance aerobics. In comparison, men are usually efficient runners. Because of anatomical differences that occur at puberty, men have wider shoulders and smaller hips; their higher center of gravity makes them more efficient runners, joggers, and athletes. Whatever body composition or anatomical structure, participants can find an aerobic program to suit their needs.

Diet.   Dieting is as personal as exercise routines. Choosing the correct diet depends on the number of calories burned in ratio to the number of calories consumed. Weight loss only occurs when more calories are used than are eaten. The best method of weight reduction, as was already stated, is an increase in exercise without a reduction of essential foods. Nevertheless, many persons want to reduce their intake, as well as increase their output. The best diet for weight loss while exercising is, unfortunately, a choice made confusing by hundreds of pseudo-diets promising quick weight loss—each with a gimmick for a slim, beautiful body. Science has proven that fat loss is a long-term endeavor.

Some aspects of weight loss are worth scrutinizing. A group selected for a prolonged, semi-starvation diet consumed 1,000 calories a day and exercised for 2.5 hours, Table 3-6.

In the first three days of weight loss, 70 percent of the 1.8 pound daily loss was water. Not until day 11 did fat loss exceed water loss, and it was not

TABLE 3-6   Water, Protein, and Fat Loss on Starvation Diet.

	DAY 1–3	DAY 11–13	DAY 21–24
Daily weight loss	1.8 lbs.	.5 lbs	4 lbs
	70% water	19% water	0% water
	5% protein	12% protein	15% protein
	25% fat	59% fat	85% fat

until day 21 that water weight stabilized. The implications are apparent: water weight is lost quickly but fat weight is not.

Nutrition. The best diet to lose weight is the best diet to maintain weight: balanced nutrition that meets minimum daily requirements. The delicate balance of necessary nutrients—minerals, vitamins, fats, proteins, carbohydrates—cannot be sacrificed. All diets must be nutritionally sound, and must contain the essential food groups. The Department of Agriculture in 1957 divided food into four standard groups. Some years ago they expanded it to seven groups. To maintain nutritional balance, we need at least two servings a day from each group, unless advised otherwise by our physicians (Table 3-7).

An example of the seven food groups listed in a daily diet is in Table 3-8. This diet contains about 1200 to 1500 calories per day. Because weight loss involves a long-term effort, nutrition needs should never be reduced below minimum standards. As we have stated earlier, consult a physician, who will consider gender, age, and size when determining the proper number of calories for a weight loss program.

Food and the Pattern of Its Consumption

For a person who exercises, an optimum diet supplies the nutrients adequate for tissue maintenance, repair, and growth. Active, exercising men and women do not require nutrients beyond those obtained from a balanced diet. Persons who eat balanced meals of the seven food groups consume more than adequate vitamins to meet daily needs. Because vitamins can be used repeatedly in metabolic processes, the vitamin needs of athletes and active persons are not greater than requirements of sedentary persons. As individuals become more active, the need for increased energy consumption also increases, which explains why a marathon runner

TABLE 3-7 Seven Basic Food Groups.

1. Meat, fish, poultry, and cheese for essential protein
2. Green vegetables for vitamins, fiber, and minerals
3. Yellow vegetables, such as potatoes, squash, and turnips, for sources of vitamins, fibers, minerals, and complex carbohydrates.
4. Fruits for sources of vitamin C, fiber, and carbohydrates. At least one serving should be a citrus fruit.
5. Breads and cereals for fiber, vitamin B, and carbohydrates
6. Milk products essential for calcium, vitamin D, and other complex vitamins and minerals
7. One serving of linoleic acid, which is a part of butter and cooking oils. Linoleic acid, essential for certain functions of the body, has to be obtained from sources outside the body.

TABLE 3-8   A Nutritional Diet for Weight Loss.

BREAKFAST: Either ½ cup cereal, 1 egg, or 1 piece toast
1 cup milk, ½ cup cottage cheese or
½ cup plain yogurt
6 ounces fruit

SNACK: (MIDMORNING)
1 cup milk or 1 small fruit

LUNCH: Lettuce, all you want
1 tomato or celery and carrots or ½ cup green or yellow vegetables.
¾ oz. hard cheese, or ½ cup cottage cheese, or 3 oz. poultry, or fish, or
½ cup plain yogurt.
1 cup clear, nonsalted soup
1 piece bread, 1 pat butter

DINNER: 3–4 oz. lean meat (3 times week only), or poultry, or fish
½ cup green vegetables
½ cup yellow vegetables
All lettuce, celery, cauliflower, cabbage, you want.
1 cup clear, unsalted soup
1 fruit: apple, orange, ½ grapefruit, pear, peach, banana

SNACK: 1 fruit, or 1 cup milk, or 1 oz. cheese

RED MEAT: No more than 3 servings a week.
EGGS: No more than 3 per week.
WATER: Drink 8 oz. glass 8 times a day.

This diet contains an excellent distribution of the seven food groups, along with low calorie intake. No fried foods, no sauces are to be added.

---

may consume as many as 5,000 calories a day. Here is the recommended nutrient intake for an active adult.

Protein. The standard recommendation for protein intake is 0.8 grams of protein per kilogram of body weight. One kg. is equal to 2.2 lbs, therefore a 130—pound person needs 47.2 grams of protein, which is one medium serving of meat. A 170 lb. person would require about 62 grams (2.19 oz.) of the total calories in the average American's diet. Unfortunately, we eat about twice as much protein as we need, and the surplus does not increase muscle mass—the additional calories are converted to fat and may add digestive strain on the liver and kidneys.

Fats. Optimal fat intake has not been firmly established, though it is believed that not more than 30 percent of the calories consumed should be fat. Of course, individuals with gall bladder disease and cardiovascular disease should avoid even this level. Too low a fat consumption can, however, decrease vitamin absorption by the body because fat-soluble vitamins must enter the body through fat consumption—essential fatty acid, linoleic acid. So a fat-free diet is potentially dangerous.

Carbohydrates.   Carbohydrates should be at least 50 to 60 percent of calorie ingestion. Carbohydrate—rich foods such as grains, starchy roots, and dried peas and beans seem to benefit those who eat them. Populations that subsist chiefly on carbohydrates, provided that essential amino acids, minerals, and vitamins are also present, have lower incidences of hypertension, obesity, constipation, and death from cardiac and circulatory complications, and colon cancer.

Fiber.   Fiber is that part of fruits, vegtables, and whole grains that our bodies cannot absorb—some is found in all plant food, but almost none is found in meat, fish, poultry, or dairy products. (Bran is probably the high-fiber food with which we are most familiar). In this fast-food world, very few persons get enough fiber. The effects of a low-fiber diet can cause constipation, hemorrhoids, colitus, diverticulum diseases, and other anal and colon disease. The time required to pass food from intake to elimination for average Americans is about two or three days. In the Orient the fecal transit time is 24 hours—because their diets are rich in fiber and carbohydrates. In America, transit times for senior citizens can be as long as two weeks. Though Americans have longer transfer times, it does not mean laxatives are needed, it simply means more fruits, grains, and vegetables should be eaten.

Fiber and its components work as a sponge to absorb water, making softer stools and easier elimination (many laxatives are based on fiber preparations). Besides relieving constipation, high-fiber diets are known to be helpful in the treatment of various digestive diseases. Additionally, a diet high in fiber can cause a three-to four-pound weight loss.

Many persons do not eat fibrous foods because they fear the additional calories of a high-carbohydrate diet. It is true that high-fiber diets are also high-carbohydrate diets. However, a diet rich in carbohydrates and fiber keeps blood-sugar levels stable throughout the day, thereby reducing the ups and downs that lead to midmorning or midafternoon sluggishness and irritability. Adding a piece of whole-grain bread, potato, or apple (with its skin), reduces the sharp changes in blood-sugar levels that do occur with a piece of apple pie, pastry, or candy. When blood-sugar levels remain stable throughout the day, being tired or hungry will not occur between meals. Calories are saved because the desire to reach for a high-calorie snack is decreased.

A high-carbohydrate, high-fiber diet helps weight loss, reduces blood-cholesterol levels, and prevents constipation, or more serious bowel disorders by providing bulk in the diet. High-fiber foods can lower cholesterol by increasing high-density lipoproteins (HDL)—a combination of a fat and protein, which acts as a scavenger to remove cholesterol from arterial walls. High-fiber foods also decrease low-density lipoproteins (LDL) that clog the arteries, and reduce cholesterol that may coat the arterial walls.

Recommended Caloric and Fiber Consumption

The nutrition committee of the American Heart Association advised Americans to increase their calories obtained from carbohydrates from 45 to 55 percent of their total, and to reduce their daily calories derived from fats from 40 percent to a maximum of 30 percent. The committee also stated that saturated fats (meat, butter, whole milk, cream, ice cream, hard cheese, vegetable oils, coconut oil, palm oil, cocoa, hydrogenated margarine, and shortening) unquestionably raise the level of cholesterol in the blood; that high blood cholesterol can directly contribute to arteriosclerosis; and that in turn increases the risk of coronary heart disease.

The latest research indicates that the body needs about 20 to 40 grams of fiber a day—nearly twice what most Americans eat. A few studies have shown that for some persons, eating large amounts of whole grains over a period of time may result in borderline deficiencies of calcium and iron. Phytate, a substance found in grains, tends to bind with these minerals, making them unavailable for use by the body. Normally, however, increasing fiber as part of a balanced diet should not present problems. Table 3-9 is a list of fibrous foods with their fiber amounts.

Monitoring Caloric Intake

If the participant is now convinced that weight loss is a good idea, and their physician has agreed, it is time to begin monitoring caloric intake.

Food and its consumption patterns can provide information about why the participant is overweight—usually the cause is too much food, too often, without sufficient exercise. Studies show that persons who exercise strenuously have built-in appetite controls. Their internal control regulates exactly how much must be consumed. Unfortunately, few of us exercise to such extremes and therefore our appetites are not curbed: our bodies tell us that we are hungry when we are not. Controlling the amount of food that we eat is learned behavior. A participant with a weight problem must modify the eating pattern.

Most Americans eat far too much fried, fatty food. Only a small part of our population eats the balanced, seven-food group each day. Even fewer persons eat in regular patterns. Most of us skip breakfast, consume a light lunch, then eat a hearty dinner, followed by snacks until bedtime. Some experts believe that all calories should be consumed before 5:00 p.m. The theory is that all calories taken after that time are not burned at the same rate as those consumed during daily activity because after dinner most of us either read, watch television, or sleep. Whether the theory is

TABLE 3-9   Dietary Fiber in Selected Common Foods.

FOOD	PORTION	DIETARY FIBER
Cereals		
White Bread	1 slice	0.7 gms.
Oatmeal (cooked)	1 cup	1.4 gms.
Whole Wheat Bread	1 slice	2.4 gms.
Bran Flakes	1 cup	4.8 gms.
All-Bran	¾ cup	12.0 gms.
Fruit		
Apple	½ medium	2.0 gms.
Cherries	1 cup	2.0 gms.
Peach	1 medium	2.1 gms.
Orange	1 medium	2.3 gms.
Raisins	¼ cup	2.3 gms.
Strawberries	1 cup	3.1 gms.
Vegetables		
Lettuce	1 cup	1.1 gms.
Tomato (raw)	1 small	1.5 gms.
Potato (baked)	½ medium	1.9 gms.
Carrots (raw)	1, 7½"	2.3 gms.
Popcorn, popped	3 cups	3.0 gms.
Peas (cooked)	½ cup	6.2 gms.
Spinach (cooked)	½ cup	6.3 gms.
Kidney beans	½ cup	7.4 gms.
Lima beans	½ cup	8.3 gms.
Broccoli (cooked)	1 cup	11.5 gms.

Recommended Daily Intake is 20-40 gms.

correct or not, there are some good points to remember: do not eat the majority of calories after 5:00 p.m., when the energy is unneeded. Eat a balanced breakfast. Blood-sugar levels affect the ability to function; if we do not eat breakfast, we will run out of energy before noon. The best breakfast is one with the basic food groups. Eat a lunch that is balanced, as well. Eat a light supper, then control the snacks by choosing a fruit or a raw vegetable, rather than sweets or potato chips.

Now that we have an estimate of percentage of fat (with an error factor of about 3 to 5 percent), we can examine eating patterns and food preference. Most individuals have weight problems because they either eat too much or exercise too little. We recommend that aerobic dance partici-pants begin to monitor their eating habits and food intake. We usually assign our participants a three-to five-day calorie monitoring. This assign-ment:

1. helps them become aware of their dietary patterns
2. makes them aware of the types and kinds of food that they eat.

If a computer is available, some good dietary analysis packages are available that will compute all calories quickly and simply.

On the following pages are lists of foods and calories. The participant keeps record of all foods ingested and determines the amount of calories consumed. By analyzing the types of foods, the instructor may be able to help the participant realize the problem areas (Table 3-10).

TABLE 3-10   Caloric Values of Selected Foods.

FOOD	SERVING	CAL
Apple, baked	1 medium, 2½ in. dia.	120
Apple, brown betty	½ cup	175
Apple juice (sweet cider)	½ cup bottle or canned	60
Apples, raw	1, (about 3 per lb.)	70
Applesauce, canned, sweetened	½ cup	115
Apricots, fresh raw (as purchased)	3 (above 12 per lb.)	55
Apricots, canned, syrup pack	½ cup or 4 medium halves, 2 tbsp. juice	110
Apricots, dried, stewed	½ cup (scant) or 8 halves 2 tbsp. juice, sweetened	135
Asparagus, cooked, green	½ cup, 1½ to 2 in. lengths	15
Avocado, raw (as purchased)	½ avocado, 3⅛ in. dia., pitted and peeled	185
Bacon, broiled or fried	2 slices, cooked crisp (20 slices per lb., raw)	90
Bacon, Canadian, cooked	3 slices, cooked crisp	100
Bananas, raw (as purchased)	1 medium	100
Bean sprouts, mung, cooked	½ cup drained	18
Beans, green lima, dry, cooked	¾ cup	195
Beans, green snap, cooked	½ cup	15
Beans, red kidney, dry, canned	¾ cup	173
Beans, white, dry, canned with tomato sauce, w/o pork	¾ cup	233
Beef, corned, canned	3 slices, 3 × 2 × ¼ in.	185
Beef, corned hash, canned	½ cup (approx.)	155
Beef, dried or chipped	4 thin slices, 4 × 5 in.	115
Beef, hamburger, broiled	1 patty, 3 in. dia. (reg. gnd.)	245
Beef potpie, baked	1 pie, 4¼ in. dia.	560
Beef, pot roast, cooked	1 piece, 4 × 3¾ × ½ in.	245
Beef roast, oven-cooked	2 slices, 6 × 3¼ × ⅛ in.	165
Beef steak, broiled, med. fat, no bone	1 piece, 3½ × 2 × ¾ in.	330
Beef stroganoff, cooked	½ cup	250
Beets, cooked	½ cup, diced	28
Beverages, cola-type	about ¾ cup	75
Beverages, ginger ale	1 cup	75
Biscuits, baking powder (enriched flour)	1 biscuit, 2 in. dia.	105
Blackberries, raw	½ cup	45

TABLE 3-10 (continued)

FOOD	SERVING	CAL
Bouillon cubes	1 cube, ⅝ in.	5
Bran flakes, 40% bran (thiamine and iron added)	¾ cup	80
Bread, Boston brown	1 slice, 3 × ¾ in.	100
Bread, cracked wheat	1 slice, 18 slices per lb. loaf	65
Bread, Italian (enriched flour)	1 slice, 3¼ × 2 × 1 in.	55
Bread, light rye (⅓ rye, ⅔ wheat)	1 slice, 18 slices per lb. loaf	60
Bread, white soft crumb (enriched)	1 slice, 18 slices per lb. loaf	70
Bread, whole wheat, firm crumb	1 slice, 18 slices per lb. loaf	60
Bread crumbs	¼ cup, dry grated	98
Broccoli, cooked	½ cup, stalks cut into ½-in. pieces	20
Brussels sprouts, cooked	½ cup or 5 medium	28
Butter	1 tbsp. or ⅛ stick	100
Cabbage, cooked short time in little water	½ cup	15
Cake, angel food (from mix)	1 piece, 1/12 of 10-in. dia. cake	135
Cake, Boston cream pie (unenriched flour)	1 piece, 1/12 of 8-in. dia. pie	210
Cake, fruit, dark (enriched flour)	1 slice, 1/30 of 8-in.-long loaf	55
Cake, plain chocolate iced cupcake (from mix)	1 cupcake, 2½ in. dia.	130
Cake, plain uniced cupcake (from mix)	1 cupcake, 2½ in. dia.	90
Cake, pound (unenriched flour)	1 slice, 2¾ × 3 × ⅝ in.	140
Cake, sponge (unenriched)	1 slice, 1/12 of 10-in. dia. cake	145
Cake, two-layer devil's food with chocolate icing (from mix)	1 slice, 1/16 of 9-in. dia. cake	235
Cake, two-layer white with chocolate icing	1 slice, 1/16 of 9-in. dia. cake	250
Candy, caramels	4 small	115
Candy, plain chocolate	1 bar, 3¾ × 1½ × ¼ in.	145
Candy, chocolate with almonds	1 bar, 5⅓ × 1⅞ × ⅓ in.	265
Candy, chocolate fudge	1 piece, 1¼ × 1¼ × 1 in.	115
Candy, hard	6 pieces, 1 in. dia., ¼ in. thick	110
Candy, peanut brittle	1 piece, 3¼ × 2½ × ¼ in.	125
Cantaloupes	½, 5 in. dia.	60
Carrots, cooked	½ cup diced	23
Carrots, raw	½ cup grated	23
Catsup, tomato (see tomato)		

TABLE 3-10 (continued)

FOOD	SERVING	CAL
Cauliflower, cooked	½ cup flowerets	13
Celery, raw	½ cup, diced	8
Celery, raw whole	1 stalk, large outer, 8 in. long	5
Cheese, cheddar (American)	1 cube, 1⅛ in.	115
Cheese, cheddar (American)	1 tbsp. grated	30
Cheese, cream	1 tbsp.	60
Cheese, creamed cottage (made from skim milk)	¼ cup	65
Cheese, Swiss (domestic)	1 slice, 7 × 4 ″ ⅛ in.	105
Cheesecake	1, ⅒ of 9-in. dia. cake	400
Cherries, raw, sweet	1 cup with stems	80
Cherries, raw, West Indian (acerola)	2 medium	3
Chicken, broiled	3 slices, flesh only	115
Chicken, canned	⅓ cup boned meat	170
Chicken, creamed	½ cup	220
Chicken breast, fried	½ breast with bone	155
Chicken drumstick, fried	1 drumstick with bone	90
Chicken pie (see poultry potpie)		
Chili con carne with beans, canned	¾ cup	250
Chili con carne w/o beans, canned	¾ cup	383
Chocolate, bitter (baking chocolate)	1 square	145
Chocolate candy (see candy)		
Chocolate-flavored milk drink (made with skim milk)	1 cup	190
Chocolate morsels	30 morsels or 1½ tbsp.	80
Chocolate syrup	2 tbsp.	80
Chop suey, cooked	¾ cup	325
Clams, canned	½ cup or 3 medium clams	45
Cocoa, beverage (made with milk)	¾ cup	176
Coconut, dried, sweetened	¼ cup, shredded	85
Coconut, fresh	¼ cup, shredded	113
Coleslaw	½ cup	50
Cookies, brownies	1 piece, 1⅞ × 1⅞ × ⅝ in.	145
Cookies, chocolate chip	1 cookie, 2¼ in. diameter	60
Cookies, coconut bar chews	1 cookie, 3 × ⅞ × ⅓ in.	55
Cookies, oatmeal with raisins and nuts	1 cookie, 2⅛ in. diameter	65
Cookies, sugar, plain	1 cookie, 2½ in. diameter	40
Corn, sweet, canned	½ cup, solids and liquid	85
Corn, sweet, cooked	1 ear, 5 in. long	70
Corn muffins (enriched flour and enriched degermed meal)	1 muffin, 2⅜ in. dia.	125

TABLE 3-10 (continued)

FOOD	SERVING	CAL
Cornflakes (added nutrients)	1⅓ cup	133
Crabmeat, canned	½ cup flakes	85
Crackers, graham, plain	2 medium or 4 small	55
Crackers, saltines	2 crackers, 2 in. square	35
Cranberry juice, canned, ascorbic acid added	½ cup or 1 small glass	85
Cranberry sauce, canned	¼ cup, strained and sweetened	85
Cream half-and-half	1 tbsp.	20
Cream, heavy, whipping	1 tbsp., unwhipped (volume doubled when whipped)	55
Creamer, coffee (imitation cream)	1 tsp. powder	10
Cucumber, raw	6 slices, pared, ⅛ in. thick	5
Dessert topping whipped (low-calorie with nonfat dry milk)	2 tbsp.	17
Doughnuts, cake-type (enriched flour)	1	125
Egg, raw, boiled, or poached	1 whole egg	80
Eggs, creamed	½ cup (1 egg in ¼ cup white sauce)	190
Eggs, fried in 1 tsp. fat	1 egg	115
Eggs, scrambled, with milk and fat	1 egg	110
Egg white, raw	1 egg white	15
Egg yolk, raw	1 egg yolk	60
Fats, cooking, lard	1 tbsp. solid fat	115
Fats, cooking, vegetable	1 tbsp. solid fat	110
Fish, creamed (tuna, salmon, or other, in white sauce)	½ cup	220
Fish sticks, breaded, cooked	5 sticks, each 3.8 × 1.0 × 0.5 in.	200
Frankfurter, heated	1 frankfurter	170
French toast, fried (enriched bread)	1 slice	180
Fruit cocktail, canned with heavy syrup	½ cup	98
Gelatin, plain, dry	1 tbsp. (1 envelope)	25
Gelatin dessert, plain	½ cup, ready to eat	70
Gingerbread (from mix)	1 piece, ⅑ of 8-in. square cake	175
Grapefruit, white, canned (syrup pack)	½ cup	88
Grapefruit, white, raw (as purchased)	½ medium, 3¾ in. dia.	45
Grapefruit juice, canned, unsweetened	½ cup	50
	½ cup or 1 small glass,	50

TABLE 3-10 (continued)

FOOD	SERVING	CAL
Grapefruit juice, dehydrated crystals	½ cup or 1 small glass, prepared, ready to serve	50
Grape juice, canned	½ cup	83
Grapes, raw American-type	1 cup or 1 medium bunch	65
Greens, spinach, cooked	½ cup	20
Greens, turnip, cooked	½ cup	15
Haddock, fried	1 fillet, 4 × 2½ × ½ in.	140
Ham, boiled	1 slice, 6¼ × 3¾ × ⅛ in.	135
Ham, cured, roasted	2 slices, 5½ × 3¾ × ⅛ in.	245
Ham, luncheon, canned	2 tbsp. spiced or unspiced	165
Honey, strained	1 tbsp.	65
Ice cream, plain (factory packed)	1 container, 3 fluid oz.	95
Ice cream, plain brick	1 slice, ⅛ of qt. brick	145
Ice milk	½ cup	100
Jams, jellies, preserves	1 tbsp.	55
Kale (see greens)		
Lamb, leg, roasted lean and fat, no bone	2 slices, 3 × 3¼ × ⅛ in.	235
Lamb chop, cooked	1 thick chop with bone	400
Lemonade, (made from frozen, sweetened concentrate)	1 cup	110
Lemon juice, fresh	1 tbsp.	5
Lentils, dry, cooked	½ cup	120
Lettuce, head, raw	1 head (compact, as iceberg), 4¾ in. dia.	60
Lettuce, loose leaf, raw	2 large leaves or 4 small leaves	10
Liver, beef, fried	1 slice, 5 × 2 × ⅓ in.	130
Liver, calf, fried	1 slice, 5 × 2 × ½ in.	230
Liver, chicken, fried	3 medium	235
Liver, pork, fried	1 slice, 3¾ × 1¾ × ½ in.	225
Macaroni, cooked (enriched)	¾ cup	115
Macaroni and cheese, baked (enriched macaroni)	¾ cup	323
Mackerel, broiled	1 piece	200
Margarine (fortified with Vitamin A)	1 tbsp. or ⅛ stick	100
Marshmallows	1, 1¼ in. dia.	25
Meat loaf, beef, baked	1 slice, 3¾ × 2¼ × ¾ in.	240
Milk, dry skim (nonfat)	¼ cup powder, instant	61
Milk, dry whole	¼ cup powder	129
Milk, evaporated, canned	½ cup, undiluted and unsweetened	173
Milk, fluid, skim or buttermilk	1 cup (½ pt.)	90
Milk, fluid, whole	1 cup (½ pt.) 3.5% fat	160

TABLE 3-10 (continued)

FOOD	SERVING	CAL
Milkshake, chocolate	1 fountain size glass	420
Muffins, plain (enriched white flour)	1, 2¾ in. dia.	120
Mushrooms, canned	½ cup solids and liquid	20
Noodles, egg, cooked (enriched)	¾ cup	150
Nuts, almonds	¼ cup shelled	213
Nuts, peanuts (see peanuts, roasted)		
Nuts, pecan halves	¼ cup	185
Nuts, walnut halves, English or Persian	¼ cup	163
Oatmeal or rolled oats, cooked (regular or quick-cooking)	⅔ cup	87
Oils, salad or cooking	1 tbsp.	125
Olives, green	4 medium or 3 large	15
Olives, ripe	3 small or 2 large	15
Onions, cooked	½ cup or 5 onions, 1¼ in. dia.	30
Onions, raw	1, 2½ in. dia.	40
Onions, young green	6 small, without tops	20
Orange juice, fresh (all varieties)	½ cup or 1 small glass	55
Orange juice, canned (unsweetened)	½ cup or 1 small glass	60
Orange juice, frozen concentrate	½ cup or 1 small glass, diluted, ready to serve	60
Oranges (all commercial varieties)	1 orange, 2⅝ in. dia.	65
Oysters, raw	½ cup or 8-10 oysters	80
Oyster stew, milk	1 cup with 3-4 oysters	200
Pancakes, wheat (enriched flour)	1 griddle cake, 4 in. dia.	60
Parsley, raw	1 tbsp. chopped	trace
Parsnips, cooked	½ cup	50
Peaches, canned halves or slices (syrup pack)	½ cup, solids and liquid	100
Peaches, canned whole (water pack)	½ cup, solids and liquid	38
Peaches, raw sliced, fresh or frozen	½ cup	33
Peaches, raw whole	1 peach, 2 in. dia.	35
Peanut butter	2 tbsp.	190
Peanuts, roasted, salted	¼ cup halves	210
Pears, canned (syrup pack)	2 med. halves with 2 tbsp. juice	90
Pears, raw (as purchased)	1 pear, 3 × 2½ in. dia.	100
Peas, cowpeas, dry, cooked (blackeye peas or frijoles)	½ cup	95

TABLE 3-10   (continued)

FOOD	SERVING	CAL
Peas, green, cooked	½ cup	58
Peas, split, dry, cooked	½ cup	145
Peppers, green, stuffed with meat stuffing, cooked	1 medium	200
Peppers, hot red (see chili powder)	1 tbsp.	20
Pickle relish		
Pickles, cucumber, bread and butter	6 slices, ¼ × 1½ diameter	30
Pickles, cucumber, dill	1 large, 3¾ × 1¼ in.	10
Pickles, cucumber, sweet	1, 2½ × ¾ in. dia.	20
Pie, apple (unenriched flour)	4-in. sector or ⅐ of 9-in. dia. pie	350
Pie, cherry (unenriched flour)	4-in. sector or ⅐ of 9-in. dia. pie	350
Pie, lemon meringue (unenriched flour)	4-in. sector or ⅐ of 9-in. dia. pie	305
Pie, mince (unenriched flour)	4-in. sector or ⅐ of 9-in. dia. pie	365
Pie, pumpkin (unenriched flour)	4-in. sector or ⅐ of 9-in. dia. pie	275
Pineapple, canned crushed (syrup pack)	½ cup	100
Pineapple, canned slices (syrup pack)	1 large or 2 small slices, 2 tbsp. juice	90
Pineapple, raw	½ cup, diced	38
Pineapple juice, canned	½ cup or 1 small glass	68
Pizza (cheese) pie	5½ in. sector or ⅛ of 14-in. dia.	185
Plums, canned (syrup pack)	½ cup or 3 plums with 2 tbsp. juice	100
Plums, raw	1 plum, 2 in. diameter	25
Popcorn, popped	1 cup (oil and salt) added	40
Pork chop, cooked	1 thick chop, trimmed with bone	260
Pork roast, cooked	2 slices, 5 × 4 × ⅛ in.	310
Potato chips	10 medium chips, 2 in. dia.	115
Potatoes, baked	1 medium, about 3 per pound raw	90
Potatoes, boiled, peeled before boiling	1	80
Potatoes, french fried cooked in deep fat	10 pieces, 2 × ½ × ½ in.	155
Potatoes, mashed	½ cup (milk & butter added)	95
Poultry (chicken or turkey) potpie	1 indiv. pie, 4¼ in. dia.	535
Pretzels	5, 3⅛ in. thick sticks	10
Prune juice, canned	½ cup or 1 small glass	100
Prunes, dried, cooked	5 medium with 2 tbsp. juice, sweetened	160

TABLE 3-10   (continued)

FOOD	SERVING	CAL
Pudding, chocolate	½ cup	190
Pudding, cornstarch (plain blanc mange)	½ cup	140
Pudding, rice with raisins (old fashioned)	½ cup	300
Pudding, tapioca	½ cup	140
Radishes, raw	4 small	5
Raisins, seedless	1 tbsp. pressed down	30
Raspberries, raw, red	½ cup	35
Rice, puffed (nutrients added)	1 cup	60
Rice flakes (nutrients added)	1 cup	115
Rolls, bagel (egg)	1 roll, 3 in. diameter	165
Rolls, barbecue bun (enriched)	1 bun, 3½ in. dia.	120
Rolls, hard	1 round roll	160
Rolls, plain, white (enriched flour)	1 commercial pan roll	85
Rolls, sweet, pan	1 roll	135
Salad, chicken, with mayonnaise	½ cup	280
Salad, egg, with mayonnaise	½ cup	190
Salad, fresh fruit (orange, apple, banana, grapes), with French dressing	½ cup	130
Salad, jellied, vegetable, no dressing	½ cup	70
Salad, lettuce, with French dressing	¼ solid head	80
Salad, potato, with mayonnaise	½ cup	185
Salad, tomato aspic, no dressing	½ cup	45
Salad, tuna fish, with mayonnaise	½ cup	250
Salad dressing, blue cheese	1 tbsp.	75
Salad dressing, boiled	1 tbsp. home-made	25
Salad dressing, commercial	1 tbsp. mayonnaise-type	65
Salad dressing, French	1 tbsp.	65
Salad dressing, low calorie	2 tbsp. (cottage cheese nonfat dry milk, no oil)	17
Salad dressing, mayonnaise	1 tbsp.	100
Salad dressing, Thousand Island	1 tbsp.	80
Salmon, broiled or baked	1 steak, 4 × 3 × ½ in.	200
Salmon, pink, canned	½ cup	120
Salmon loaf	½ cup or 1 slice, 4 × 1¼ × 1¼ in.	235
Sauce, chocolate	2 tbsp.	75
Spaghetti, in tomato sauce, with cheese	¾ cup	200

TABLE 3-10 (continued)

FOOD	SERVING	CAL
Spaghetti, in tomato sauce, with meat balls	¾ cup	250
Spinach (see greens)		
Squash, summer, cooked	½ cup diced	15
Squash, winter, baked	½ cup, mashed	65
Stew, beef and vegetable	¾ cup	160
Strawberries, raw	½ cup, capped	30
Sugar, brown	1 tbsp. firmly packed	50
Sugar, granulated (beet or cane)	1 tbsp.	40
Sugar, lump	1 domino, 1⅛ × ¾ × ⅜ in.	25
Waffles (enriched flour)	1 waffle, 7 in. diameter	210
Watermelon, raw	1 wedge, 4 × 8 in., with rind	115
Wheat, shredded	1 biscuit, 4 × 2¼ in.	90
Wheat flakes (nutrients added)	1 cup	105
Wheat flour, white (enriched)	1 cup sifted	420
Wheat flour, white	1 cup sifted	400
Wheat flour, whole wheat (hard wheat)	1 cup	400
Wheat germ	2 tbsp.	30
White sauce (medium)	¼ cup	110

Source: Stoll, S. *The University Fitness Guide*, 1986. Reprinted by permission: University Press, Moscow, ID.

A Sensible Diet

After monitoring the diet, the participant can begin the weight loss program. However, please remember that before any participant goes on a diet, a physician should be consulted. The participant must then make a commitment to change their eating and exercising behaviors. Weight loss and weight maintenance are lifelong endeavors that cannot be accomplished without eating properly and exercising adequately. Because of metabolic processes, weight loss does not occur overnight. If a participant wants to lose weight safely, a few rules may help.

1. A calorie is a measure of energy. Since energy enters the body as food, and leaves as heat, calories are measured in units of heat. The calorie count of food is the amount of energy it provides.
2. Energy-in should equal to energy-out. If the two are equal, weight is maintained. If the equating becomes imbalanced, weight is gained or lost.
3. Determine how many calories are needed per day for weight maintenance or weight loss. To find the caloric needs, a simple formula can be used. One calorie per hour is needed for every 2.2 pounds of body weight. A 125-pound

woman, for example, needs 1,368 calories to maintain her bodily functions. Add to that the calories expended daily by physical activity, and we have the number of calories needed to maintain weight. An easier formula for a moderately-active woman is to multiply weight by 15.

4. Cut 500 calories a day to lose one pound a week. It follows that cutting 1000 calories a day will cause a two-pound loss. Because such a large reduction is questionable, a participant should do so only with a physician's recommendation.

5. One gram of protein contains four calories, and so does one gram of carbohydrate. But one gram of fat contains nine calories. Pies, French fries, Big Macs, butter, salad dressings, and the like, contain a lot of fat grams. Eliminating them will cut more calories.

6. Adjust the calories to meet the circumstances. Caloric needs change depending on such factors as body size, pregnancy, breast feeding, amount of exercise, gender, and climate.

7. Cut calories every year. Age is an important factor in how many calories you need. It is presently thought that basal metabolism slows due to the aging process. Some research indicates that the reduced metabolic rate is due to a sedentary lifestyle. If individuals would continue to exercise vigorously, perhaps metabolic rate would not decrease.

8. No diet is complete without exercise. If we diet without exercising we lose more protein mass and less fat tissue; conversely, by combining exercise with diet, we lose more fat than protein.

9. Exercise must accompany any attempt to lose weight. Although exercise is a requisite for weight loss, it is not the answer for gross overeating or binging. Diets too rich in calories, unaccompanied by sufficient exercise, result in excess fat. The chart below clearly illustrates how much exercise it takes to burn the excess calories of rich food (Table 3-11).

10. There is no such thing as spot reducing. Weight cannot be reduced in one particular area. Fat must be oxidized throughout the whole body. We can, however, tone muscles in one area, thereby reducing the intramuscular fat and building the muscle. Since muscle is more dense than fat, the area will become smaller in girth. Storage fat cannot be reduced in one area without affecting storage fat throughout the body.

TABLE 3-11   Caloric Cost Equated with Selected Foods.

FOOD	CAL.	MIN. OF WALKING	MIN. OF BICYCLING	MIN. OF SWIMMING	MIN. OF RUNNING
Beer	115	22	18	14	6
Cola	105	20	16	12	6
Plain Donut	164	32	25	19	9
Chocolate Bar	198	38	30	23	11
Spaghetti	295	57	45	35	16
Chocolate Chip Cookies	150	29	23	18	8
Ice Cream Cone	160	31	25	19	9
Hamburger Plain	224	43	34	26	12

11. Weight charts distributed by insurance companies are not accurate indicators of a desirable weight.
12. When dieting, participants should remember to eat the proper balance of nutritional foods. They should not give up necessary vitamins, minerals, protein, carbohydrates, and lineolic acid for the benefits of exercise or for excessive weight loss. They should remember to eat moderately, but correctly.
13. Artificial devices like massage machines cannot bring about weight loss. Fat cannot be rolled or shaken off. Massage does help circulation and relieves tension, but weight can only be lost through oxidation.

A Final Note About Weight Control and Obesity

The most important object for any individual in a weight loss program is fitness. As instructors, our task is to promote the six components of health-related fitness. The most important object for any individual in a weight loss program is fitness. As instructors, our task is to promote the six components of health-related fitness: cardiovascular efficiency, muscular strength and endurance, flexibility, weight control, good nutrition, and stress reduction. Be careful that participants who are concerned about weight loss do not become obsessive. Anorexia and bulimia are results of obsessions about weight control.

STRESS REDUCTION

Becoming fit through the components of health-related fitness can alleviate or reduce stress, the sixth component of health-related fitness. Stress is one of the most debilitating medical and social problems in our country today. The President's Commission on Mental Health reported that:

1. as many as 25 percent of all Americans suffer the ill effects of excessive stress,
2. the majority of Americans die from illnesses that could be stress-related; and
3. approximately 50 percent of all general medical practice patients are suffering from stress-related problems.

Some authorities believe that as many as 70 percent of general medical problems are results of stress.

Specifically, stress is our body's response to any demand. Stress response probably is an ancient biological relic that we have inherited from our primitive ancestors. It is an arousal mechanism that nature uses to prepare the human body for physical action. This physical action can be manifested in either a fight-or-flight response.

The stress response begins at the moment we are exposed to a stressor: any person, place, or thing that ultimately causes us to experience a stress response. There are two basic classes of stressors: (1) sympathomimetic stressors, and (2) psychosocial stressors.

Sympathomimetic Stressors

Sympathomimetic stressors are chemicals that mimic our sympathetic nervous system's fight-or-flight response. Sympathomimetic stressors belong to a family of drugs known as *xanthines*, which are powerful stimulants. A typical xanthine is caffeine found in chocolate, colas, and tea.

Coffee is the most common and widely consumed source of caffeine in this country. Americans over the age of 14 consume an average of three cups of coffee a day. A six-once cup of coffee contains about 108 milligrams of caffeine. Consumption of more than 250 milligrams per day is excessive and can have adverse effects on the human body, such as anxiety, irritability, diarrhea, arrhythmias (irregular heart beats), and an inability to concentrate, in addition to a host of other stress-response symptoms. Ingesting twenty cups of coffee all at once could be lethal.

Sympathomimetic stressors cause a stress response just by consuming them. Obviously if we want to reduce stress, we should eliminate or reduce consumption of sympathomimetic stressors.

Psychosocial Stressors

A psychosocial stressor is any person, place, or thing that causes stress because of the way in which we have interpreted that person, place, or thing. In this case, it is not the stressor that causes our stress response, rather it is our perception of that stressor. A psychosocial stressor becomes a stressor by virtue of the fact that we interpreted some person, place, or thing as perhaps threatening, challenging, or in some way aversive.

Physiological Response to Stress

Once we experience stress, the hypothalamus (a small central section of the brain that regulates body temperature, certain metabolic processes, and hormone secretions), fires off information to three ductless endocrine glands (adrenal medulla, adrenal cortex, and the thyroid gland) to secrete stress hormones.

Once the stress hormones are released into the blood, they activate three major organ systems in the human body: the muscular system, the gastrointestinal system, and the cardiovascular system.

Muscle Response.   Muscles are our only means of expression. We use muscles for speech, facial expression, eye movements, every mode of expression and of feeling, and every resolution of an emotion. No matter how hard we try to hide our feelings, muscles give us away. Classic muscular response to stress include clenched teeth and frowning accompanied by tightened neck muscles. We may even assume a hunched-over posture, as if we are ready to attack, while clenching our fists and bending our arms.

A prolonged response to stress brings about chronically tense muscles that complete a feedback loop and further stimulate the mind which results in more stress. Chronically tense muscles result in numerous psycho-somatic disorders, including headache, backache, spasms of the esophagus and colon (the latter resulting in either diarrhea or constipation) posture problems, asthma, tightness in the throat and chest, eye problems, lockjaw, muscle tears and pulls, and perhaps rheumatoid arthritis.

Gastrointestinal System.   Unlike the muscular system, the gastroin-testinal system hides its stress arousal very well, at least from others. But the stress has an insipid effect, and the result is loss of appetite, a gnawing feeling in the pit of the stomach, and nausea. Continual response will result in ulcers.

Cardiovascular System.   One of the most commonly researched effects of stress arousal is high blood pressure, or hypertension. It has been esti-mated that perhaps 15 to 20 percent of our adult population suffers from blood pressure above 160/95. The World Health Organization states that a blood pressure of 140/90 or above for a prolonged period of time is consid-ered hypertensive. (Normal blood pressure for men is typically 120/70 and for women about 100/60 to 120/60). Approximately 90 percent of these cases are essential hypertension, which means they are of unknown origin. Blood pressure is the pressure exerted by the blood on the blood vessel walls. Since the primary work of the heart is to overcome the pressure in the arteries to which the blood must flow, increasing blood pressure greatly increases the work of the heart and contributes to cardiovascular disease.

Like the heart, the blood vessels have an inherent muscle tone that can be altered moment-to-moment by both the central nervous system and adrenal hormones. Anticipation and states such as fear, anger, and anxiety will constrict the vessels, thus increasing blood pressure; higher blood pres-sure is a physical response to symbolic or imagined threats: the fight-or-flight response.

Another problem with hypertension is the destruction of coronary vessels by the infusion of fatty plaques. As discussed in Chapter 2, the result of plaque build-up is atherosclerosis. The relationship between stress and blood vessel disease appears to lie in the hormones epinephrine and cortisol which mobilize fats and cholesterol for use by the muscles. These fats and cholesterol circulate in the bloodstream until used or reabsorbed. Although there are other factors in developing atheriosclerosis, constantly saturating the system with unneeded fats because of the stress reponse only exacerbates the problem. The arteriole plaque lining contains cholesterol, triglycerides, and other fats. An artery infused with such plaques will even-tually lose elasticity and harden, producing the disease arteriosclerosis (an

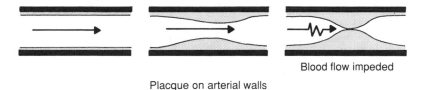

Blood flow impeded

Placque on arterial walls

advanced form of atherosclcrosis), which is directly responsible for over one-half million deaths annually in America (Figure 3-1).

When an artery is in the advanced stages of arteriosclerosis, the loss of elasticity causes blood pressure to elevate, thus contributing to hypertension and heart disease. These plaques narrow the diameter of blood vessels and diminish oxygen delivery, which may precipitate a myocardial infarction (or heart attack) if the coronary arteries are involved.

Exercise and Stress Reduction

Aerobic exercise can be a major factor in reducing the chances of plaque build-up on arteriole walls. As you remember from Chapter 2, aerobic exercise increases high density lipoproteins which act a scavengers to remove plaque from arteriole walls. At the same time, aerobic exercise decreases very-low density and low-density lipoproteins which are the fat carrying molecules. Therefore, by aerobically exercising, we can help reduce hypertension by removing plaque and by reducing our storage fat percentages.

In addition to physiologically helping hypertension, exercise also has an effect on the psychosocial aspect of the stress response. In several studies exercise has been shown to reduce stress. In one study at a major university, fifty-eight men were put into a physical fitness program, which included three ninety-minute workout sessions, three times a week. At each session the participants jogged for ten minutes to warm up, did calisthenics for twenty-five minutes, jogged for twenty-five minutes, and engaged in a recreational physical activity for twenty-five minutes. In addition to certain changes in body chemistry as a result of becoming more physically fit, the participants in this study showed increased self-assurance with their overall fitness. Another study of forty-eight university students who had experienced "test anxiety," or stress and tension before and during written exams, showed similar benefits in reducing anxiety through meditative relaxation techniques and aerobic exercise. Apparently, jogging combined with a relaxation program is an appropriate prescriptive treatment for high-anxiety individuals.

Stress reduction has been found to be essential in an overall program of health-related fitness. A weekly program of aerobic exercise combined with learning how to manage stress is imperative for overall fitness.

A Final Note About Stress Reduction

Reduction of stress is as individual as the color of our eyes. Stress management, therefore, must be an individual, personalized experience. What helps us manage stress may not help anyone else. What is important to remember is that a personalized exercise program can help in managing stress response. Education about the scientific knowledge of exercise, its effect on the sixth component of health-related fitness, and an active exercise routine will help the aerobic dance participant enjoy life so much more.

chapter

4

Education of Health-Related Fitness in the Aerobic Dance Program

INTRODUCTION

As we stated in Chapter 1, we believe that information about fitness must be disseminated to the aerobic dance participant. We do realize that many participants complain if too much exercise time is directed toward lecture. To meet the value of education demands creativity if the instructor is to present cognitive fitness material to participants.

USING EDUCATION TO HELP PARTICIPANTS LEARN

Visual Aids

One creative method is using a VCR (Video Cassette Recorder) to make a video concerning fitness components and correct training procedures, such as training effects, overload, specificity, and so forth. Once the tape is made, participants watch either on their own before class or sometime during the six to ten week exercise period. In fact, tapes could be checked-out so that participants could view at their leisure. This educational method is highly effective as long as participants are motivated to view the tapes. To ensure that participants understand the fitness information, an evaluative procedure needs to be developed. A question and answer period to review the information could be incorporated. Or possibly, a pen and pencil quiz could be administered with the reward of a cost-free exercise session or minutes toward a free session given for good scores.

A second effective method to present information related to fitness is through handouts. Fitness information concerning strength, flexibility, cardiovascular efficiency, diet, nutrition, stress reduction, and training techniques can be printed and distributed to every participant. However, the participant, unless motivated, will probably ignore the information. Obviously, the educational material must be an important part of the program and referred to often if participants are to become knowledgeable about fitness. Develop a similar assessment technique as used in the VCR teaching program to evaluate participants' knowledge.

Perhaps the educational information can be presented through classroom lecture before beginning the aerobic exercise protocol. This technique works quite well. However, the instructor must be enthusiastic and organized. Participants will not accept boring lectures that take time from their exercise period. Give 5 to 7 minute information briefs concerning fitness before each 60-minute class. If the lectures are not stimulating and interesting, many participants will avoid the first 5 to 7 minute exercise period and feel that they did not miss *a thing*. Avoid taking time away from their exercise period. In addition, a motivational technique should be developed to assess their knowledge. Do not underestimate participants' acceptance of evaluative techniques. If the program is approached with creative, positive perspectives, participants will learn.

Whatever method is used to disseminate information, remember that education is extremely important. If the instructor is committed to exercise, the participants will become committed. The greatest compliment for an aerobic dance teacher is to have students exercise on their own. We develop audio cassettes specifically for that purpose (See Chapter 9, for concerns about copyright laws.) We want our participants to learn and be motivated to perform aerobics on their own. They have learned good training techniques and the principles of fitness. They understand the components of fitness and practice them. Of course, if participants are educated, they may not return to your class, which is difficult for business. Some participants will leave but more will enroll, because they will hear about a quality program. Be positive and teach educational principles relative to fitness.

APPLYING SCIENCE IN DEVELOPING A SAFE PROGRAM

Unfortunately, many programs with incompetent exercise instructors violate training principles. Incompetency is usually linked to poor or limited training. This usually occurs because instructors cannot commit adequate time to learn new information, and therefore use unqualified sources such as commercial video tapes as their reference sources. Sometimes aerobic dance instructors want us to teach them everything we know in two weeks—a rather difficult assignment considering our years of formal education and practical experience. We give them as much information as possible but this is still not enough to become adequately knowledgeable relative to fitness. This is true of all aerobic dance seminars or continuing education programs. The clinic instructor usually has current knowledge but cannot teach everything she knows in a short span of time. The best method to gain current fitness knowledge is to enroll in exercise science classes at a local college or university. If this is not possible, become certified through a responsible agency, and enroll in an ACSM (American College of Sport Medicine) Exercise Leader/Aerobics Certification (more about that in Chapter 9). Third, attempt to keep abreast of current information from competent sources. Finding competent sources is difficult. The best advice is to learn as much as possible from sources with valid credentials.

Pre-exercise Screening

Developing a safe and efficient program is contingent on a pre-exercise screening program. Many individuals have physical disabilities that should exclude their participation in aerobic dance. Aerobic dance is a potentially dangerous activity. The joint stress of a three-day-a-week program is equal to that of running 9 to 18 miles a week. Cardiovascular stress has the potential of causing cardiac arrest. No one should be in aerobic dance without understanding the injury potential and no one 35 years or older should participate in aerobic dance without a medical screening, including a graded exercise stress test.

As we mentioned earlier, physiological function decreases with age, so older participants are unable to perform as well as younger ones. Unfortunately, most people refuse to accept the aging phenomenon. People are saturated with media "hype" about being young and beautiful. Most people attempt to find that fountain of youth. If a participant gains a few pounds or becomes unfit, he joins an exercise club and attempts to right the wrong. The exercise leader is always a young, beautiful person who encourages everyone to "go for the burn," "get with it," "lift those legs," and so on. However, most unfit people do not perform or function as well as those young, fit instructors. Each participant is an individual. The older a participant becomes, the slower their bodies become. People cannot work as hard as they did when they were 19 years old, because the aging process begins approximately at age 21. After 30 the aging process becomes more pronounced, and by the time individuals are 50, they finally become aware that changes are occurring. However, aging does not mean that a person is over the hill. Aging only means that participants should be sensible, follow acceptable exercise guidelines, and realize the age-related changes.

Physical examinations that include a blood screening and an exercise stress test are recommended after age 35. The blood analysis gives information concerning blood lipid content. As you remember, blood lipids are the fat content within the circulation system. Exercise has a tendency to increase high density lipoproteins—good blood lipids. Unfortunately, sedentary populations have increased levels of LDLs, which clog arterial walls by clinging to the lining of the vascular system. LDLs are prime factors in atheriosclerosis and cardiac disease.

The exercise stress test, discussed in Chapter 1, examines the heart, lungs, and vascular system while in a state of work. The physician or assistant monitors heart rate and blood pressure at incremental stages during the test. If any abnormalities occur, the physician is able to diagnose them. Many women are informed that as long as they are in the age range to bear children, menses will protect them from heart attacks. That is somewhat statistically true because menstruating women seldom suffer heart attacks, but the possibility still exists. Fortunately, medicine has made rapid progress in the last few decades. If a physician does diagnose signs of heart disease, many medications and advanced surgical techniques can treat those abnormalities. The stress test should be viewed as another means to evaluate a participant's exercise level.

Pre-Exercise Evaluation Form

Participants in aerobic dance programs should be required to complete an exercise and fitness evaluation form. The purpose is to screen any potential health problems before participants enter a program, as well as to avoid potential lawsuits, later (see Chapter 8: Legal Liability). Keep in mind that anyone can file a lawsuit against another person or firm. All that is required is to prepare a complaint and file it with a court, together with the required filing fee. The person filing the complaint usually tries to show that the instructor was incompetent or negligent. However, negligence can be partially averted through showing concern for the physiological functioning of each participant before they enroll in a dance exercise program. Typical questions to ask in a pre-exercise screening include:

1. Has your doctor ever said you have heart trouble?
2. Do you frequently have pains in your heart and chest?
3. Do you often feel faint or have spells of severe dizziness?
4. Has a doctor ever said your blood pressure was too high?
5. Has your doctor ever told you that you have a bone or joint problem such as arthritis that has been aggravated by exercise, or might be made worse with exercise?
6. Is there a good physical reason not mentioned here why you should not follow an activity program if you want to?
7. Are you over age 69 and unaccustomed to vigorous exercise?

If participants answer "yes" to any of these questions, do not enroll them in an aerobic dance program. Insist that they consult a physician. Again, fervently believe in, and recommend that all participants complete a physical examination. Of course, physical examinations with stress tests are expensive and many participants will not agree to the cost. However, what is more valuable—their life or the test?

Aerobic Dance Consent Form

After determining the participant's physical condition, each should be informed of the potential problems in aerobic dance exercise. Have participants sign an Aerobic Dance Consent Form (see page 90) that informs them of these possibilities. These forms have limited legal merit (see Chapter 8: Legal Liability). However, an attorney should be hired to establish legal guidelines for any exercise program. If you are not respresented by counsel, then at least subscribe to a professional reports corporation such as: The Exercise Standards and Malpractice Reporter, 4665 Douglas Circle, N.W., Canton, Ohio 44718 ($39.95 per year/six issues), to keep abreast of current legal problems and issues in exercise practices.

Consent forms do not replace an attorney's knowledge and recommendations. The Consent form is only an instrument to reaffirm educational material relative to aerobic dance and injury potential.

Applying Science in Developing Workout Protocol

After collecting pertinent information concerning pre-exercise screening, medical releases, and educational material, develop the basic workout protocol for each aerobic dance session. Because aerobic dance is a facet of aerobic fitness, individual sessions should mirror aerobic fitness objectives: developing cardiovascular (CV) efficiency, strength, flexibility, and promoting weight control, good nutrition, and stress reduction. To accomplish all of these effectively and efficiently requires organization and creativity.

First, ensure that every session begins or focuses on good training tips. Aerobic dance participants and instructors have an insatiable desire for more information. As we stated earlier the session need only be a few minutes. After the educational session, and always keeping in mind teachable moments when more information can be disseminated, is the actual exercise program.

Aerobic dance like all aerobic exercise programs, has the following exercise components: Warm-up, Strength Building, Aerobic Exercise, Cool-down.

Aerobic Warm-up The warm-up prepares the body for exercise. The warm-up circulates blood to the limbs, warms the body by raising the body

AEROBIC DANCE CONSENT FORM

Name _____ Age ____ Gender ____ Phone _____

Address _____ City _____ State _____

Physical condition: excellent ____ good ____ fair ____ poor ____

When was your last stress test? _____

Has your physician agreed to your participation in aerobic activity?____

How often do you now participate in aerobic activity?_____

You as a participant should be aware of the nature and risks involved in aerobic activity. The class includes a progressive warm-up workout, strength building, aerobic (vigorous) exercise, flexibility, and cool-down. The workloads for all strength, flexibility and aerobic activity will be at safe and acceptable work loads of 60-80% of maximal for your age group. You will receive instruction on monitoring of cardiovascular efficiency (aerobics) as well as strength, flexibility, stress reduction, weight control and nutrition.

If you are sensible and follow the program, you should improve in all six health-related fitness components. As in any physical activity, you run the risk of injury. Acute risk of participation in a vigorous exercise program is cardiac failure. However, if your physician has approved your exercise program, the possibility of cardiac failure is improbable, but always possible. Due to such risk, you are required to follow approved physical fitness guidelines that will be given to you. Additional risks that can occur are: muscle soreness, cramping and/or strained muscles, joint sprains, stress fractures, knee cartilage or ligament damage, nausea during and after exercise, heavy breathing during and after exercise, and possible exhaustion and fatigue. However, the possibility of any of these occurring is minimal, if you follow correct exercise protocol.

Your participation in this program is voluntary and you may withdraw at any time. Your written consent indicates that you have full knowledge and understand the nature of aerobic dance, the benefits you may expect, the risks that may be encountered, and you agree to participate on that basis.

Informed Consent—Liability Disclaimer and Waiver

I have read and understand the above information and do give my approval to participate in aerobic dance. I assume all risks incidental to the conduct of the classes. I do further release, absolve, indemnify, and hold harmless the instructor, _____; facility, _____: and the sponsoring agency _____. In case of injury to myself, I hereby waive all claims against the organizers and/or instructor/s.

_____ Date   _____ Signature

_____ Parent or guardian if under 18

temperature, and readies the body for strenuous exercise through flexibility or stretching movements.

The warm-up should begin with a 3 to 5 minute *mild* locomotor activity. This mild locomotor activity, like walking, skipping, jogging, jumping jacks, and so forth, prepares the body for work and stretching activities. Stretching without a mild locomotor warm-up inhibits the body's ability to stretch. How can the body have blood supplies available for stretching if the blood has not been supplied? A colleague states that stretching without a calisthenic warm-up is like revving a cold automobile motor on a wintry morning . . . it is just asking for trouble.

Second, develop a series of flexibility stretches. Various examples of stretches are available and many are good, however, some are dangerous. Refer to Chapter 2 for stretching exercises that address the major muscles and joints. The purpose of stretching is two-fold: 1) to warm the elastic tissue of the joints and muscles, and 2) to decrease the injury potential. The duration of the flexibility warm-up is relative. Some people require 10 to 15 minutes of stretching. While others swear they do not need any warm-up and have never suffered an injury. This is possible since some individuals have an anatomical predisposition and genetic traits for ample flexibility. However, the case is not true for everyone. Some individuals are so tight that they can rupture an achilles tendon by merely walking. Risking the chance of injury is ridiculous. Take the time to warm the elastic tissue in preparation for aerobic work. Probably the best flexibility warm-up should be 10 to 15 minutes depending on the age, fitness level, and activity history.

The flexibility work, because of the anatomical construction of elastic tissue, should always be static, without dynamic movement of any type.

Strength Building. After the warm-up isolated strength building should be implemented. Strength is defined as the ability to move a resistance. As you remember, strength can be developed in one of four different ways:

1. Increased resistance by increasing the amount of weight.
2. Increase resistance by keeping weight constant but increasing the amount of repetitions.
3. Increase resistance by keeping weight constant but increasing the number of repetitions in a set period of time.
4. Increase resistance by decreasing the amount of rest time between sets or repetitions.

In an aerobic dance session, weight machines or free weights may be unavailable or require too much time to use. Also, many people cannot use weights because of the additional stress placed on the skeletal system. Strength can be developed in an aerobic dance session through alternative methods.

Any group of muscles may be targeted by isolated muscle strength or endurance exercise depending on the purpose. However, the length of the strength building session should be limited to 5 to 7 minutes.

Aerobic Dance Session.   After the warm-up and strength-building phases, the aerobic exercise session begins. An aerobic dance session should be a minimum of 20 to 30 minutes. The instructor must be organized since the total time already used is: 21 to 30 minutes: a 5-minute educational program, 3 to 5 minute mild locomotor warm-up, 10 to 15 minute warm-up, and 3 to 5 minute strength session.

The aerobic dance session should begin with a mildly vigorous routine and build to more vigorous ones. Many middle-aged participants do not realize their own limitations. They should be constantly reminded to work in their own training range and not another person's level. We recommend an extra aerobic dance instructor on the floor who monitors and corrects poor postural alignment, watches for fatigue, and acts as an on-the-spot motivator.

Many so-called "fitness professionals" state that you do not have to monitor heart rates. Rather, an instructor can watch for signs of fatigue such as rapid breathing, redness, and sweating. They believe these indicators will give approximations of fatigue level. Supposedly some people need to work harder than their age-corrected training zone because they are in such good shape.

We do not agree and we would never use such an eye-ball technique. Do not fall into this trap. Take time to monitor heart rates. Check pulses often. How often? That depends on the intensity of the aerobic dances and participant's aerobic fitness levels. Remember a 20 to 30 minute aerobic dance session at participant training intensity is important. Do not choreograph aerobic dances that force participants above their training zones. Of course, some can handle higher loads compared to others, and everyone wants to be challenged. However, be sensitive to the individual needs of group participants. Develop routines that are adaptable to different work loads and intensity levels. (See Chapter 6: Skilled as a Teacher: Part II)

The major emphasis of the pulse check is to monitor participant's training levels. If some participants complain about the waste of time, have them run in place while everyone monitors their heart rates. Keep everyone moving during the pulse check. Because the potential for blood pooling (see below) is always present, all participants should be kept walking during the pulse check.

After the aerobic exercise session, add a second strength-building session for the advanced participants. Beginners who have difficulty completing the first strength session should not do this protocol. For more advanced aerobic dancers, sets of push-ups (Figure 4-1) and sit-ups (Figure

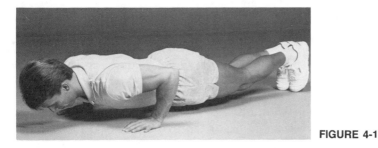

FIGURE 4-1

4-2) at the end of the session, should begin with 10 of each, then 7 of each, 5, 3 and 1. These exercises are performed without partner aid. By stressing the rectus abdominus without the feet held, the upper 4 inches of muscle is worked. In this manner, the pectoralis major, triceps, and rectus abdominus are stressed again. These sets are performed as quickly as possible, and the instructor should positively motivate so that the sets are done.

Cool-Down. Finally, we come to the cool-down phase, probably the easiest yet most important aspect of the workout. The cool-down phase returns the body to relatively normal heart rates (even though the heart rate will be elevated for up to 24 hours after a strenuous aerobic program), reduces lactic acid and fluid build-up in the muscles, and decreases the potential of blood pooling.

The phenomenon of blood pooling is an accumulation of blood in the lower extremities after intense cardiovascular work. The result is a diminished blood supply to the brain and heart. Symptoms may include: light-headedness, abnormally slow heart rate, nausea, unconsciousness, and possibly heart failure. Usually if the participant becomes too light-headed, fainting will occur. As the body assumes a horizontal position, blood returns to the heart and brain and consciousness is regained. Obviously such symptoms are extremely dangerous and all aerobic participants should follow accepted cool-down guidelines to reduce the potential of blood pooling.

FIGURE 4-2

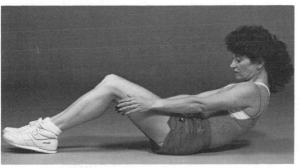

Lactic acid and fluid build-up in the muscles occur as by-products of the energy system available to supply the muscles. The exact mechanism after exercise that causes tight, sore muscles is unknown. As we discussed in Chapter 2, the soreness may occur from minute tears in the muscle fibers or increases in osmotic fluid. If the muscle is placed on stretch for one to two minutes after intense work, waste products are removed via the blood and the resultant pain and soreness are reduced. Also, by placing the muscle on stretch for one to two minutes soreness is minimized and participants will be eager to return to the next session. A little soreness is expected in untrained populations and in individuals who are striving to become stronger, but too much soreness in untrained participants will result in a low participant retention rate. If they cannot move the next day, many participants will avoid continued participation. Women in particular do not understand muscle soreness. Few unfit, adult women have a past athletic history; they have never been challenged to meet the physical demands of exercise, nor have they experienced muscle soreness.

The cool-down should incorporate light motor activities, thereby reducing the blood pooling potential in the lower extremities. Stretching the major exercise muscle groups for 1 to 2 minutes should be included. The cool-down phase should be approximately 10 minutes in duration and the participant should have recovered sufficiently to leave the exercise session with no undue fatigue or strain.

USING EDUCATION TO DEVELOP, PROVIDE, AND DEMAND ADEQUATE FACILITIES, EQUIPMENT, AND DRESS

Facilities

Adequate facilities pose a financial burden on aerobic dance facility managers as well as a legal and ethical concern for aerobic dance instructors (see Chapter 8). Adequate facilities have plenty of floor space, good ventilation, resilient flooring, acceptable acoustics, adequate sound systems, clean working showers, and a bright, cheery atmosphere. The cost to provide such facilities is quite expensive, but without acceptable facilities, the instructor as well as the participants will be at risk to incur injuries. (See Chapter 7 for discussion of injuries).

Unfortunately, many instructors provide aerobic dance classes in less than acceptable conditions, such as warehouses, fire stations, community centers, and so forth. These instructors believe that even if the facilities are poor, any exercise is better than no exercise. Little do they know that this logic is faulty.

A good aerobic experience occurs in facilities that have adequate flooring, lighting, ventilation, and so forth.

Floor Space. Since typical high impact aerobic dance choreography uses the eight locomotor movements, walk, run, jump, skip, hop, leap, glide, and gallop (See Chapter 5), each participant needs at least a 10-foot square space in which to move. Without adequate space, participants are at risk to be bumped, hit, or kicked, which may result in instant trauma (bruises, lacerations, or sprains). The floor space, as well as the accompanying wall space, should be clean and free from debris and obstacles. Dirty floors can cause the participants to slip and slide.

Research states that any type of plyometric (rebounding) exercise should be performed on a surface that has the correct amount of resiliency, stability, and durability. Resiliency is the floor's ability to absorb shock that would normally be transmitted back into the participant's feet, legs, and back. The correct amount of resiliency is one in which as the foot contacts the surface, the surface gives optimally with the impact. Surveys of injured aerobic dance participants and instructors show a possible positive linear correlation between the number of stress injuries and specific aerobic dance flooring. Naturally, instructors suffer the highest percentage of stress injuries since the longer anyone participates in aerobic dance, the greater the chance of injury on inadequate flooring. The highest stress injury rate occurs on concrete floors covered with a pad or carpet. Wood over an airspace, even with a padded carpet, also has a high stress injury rate.

Apparently, the best flooring has a resiliency factor either in the base or sub-base construction. That is, the floor has some give to it. Three varieties of flooring are recommended:

1. Suspension floor: an absorbent, resilient pad is laid first, either covering the total area, or in strips with spacing between subflooring and a finished floor covering.
2. Spring floor: coiled springs are installed proportionately apart with the sub-floor connected to the springs and topped with a finished floor.
3. Padded floor: padding of three-quarters to one inch thick is laid over a hardwood surface or concrete. The padding is of good absorbent and resilient quality and is covered with a finished floor product.

Besides resiliency, a floor must also have stability, the ability to protect instructor and participants from foot roll over and ankle turns. Concrete is the most stable surface, while foam is the least stable. However, concrete has a zero resiliency factor in contrast to foam with a high factor. A good floor has a combination of both surface stability and resiliency. Many commercial floors can provide an adequate aerobic floor.

The cost of any floor is expensive. However, the purchaser should take into account durability and what other uses the floor may provide. Of course, any of the floors can be constructed to be portable.

Ventilation.   Adequate ventilation in an exercise setting is imperative for maintaining optimal body temperatures. Unfortunately, some people think that the more they sweat during exercise, the better it is for their conditioning. This is not true. Physiologically, perspiration is a means for the body to cool itself during heavy exercise. During exercise the source of heat energy is largely in the metabolic processes of muscle tissue. Consequently, muscle temperatures during exercise are at the highest point in a gradient of temperatures. In extemely heavy, long-term activity, such as marathon running, deep-muscle temperatures have been known to rise as high as 109° F. Under the same circumstances, body-core temperatures (usually taken as rectal temperature) may be as high as 106° F, with no long-term bodily effect.

On the other hand, the temperature of the skin follows environmental temperature. During exercise in a cold environment, for example, the skin temperature may be as low as 83° F, while the core temperature is over 100° F.

In other words, muscle and core temperatures vary proportionately with the work rate and duration, while skin temperature is more related to environmental conditions. The rise in body temperature that occurs in exercise is due to a physiological readjustment of the setting of the body's "thermostat" that is entirely beneficial in that it allows muscle function to occur at higher, more efficient temperatures.

The mechanism involved in "resetting" the body's thermostat is not yet known, but it could be a result of nervous reflexes, circulating metabolites, or elaboration of hormones.

Since exercise results in increased heat production, and since the core temperature levels off and remains constant even at a new, higher level, heat dissipation must increase to maintain balance. Heat dissipation can occur in the human body by four means: (1) conduction, (2) convection (3) radiation, and (4) vaporization. Ordinarily, conduction, heat dissipating from one body to another, is unimportant since so little heat is lost. However, at rest, under moderate climatic conditions, most metabolic heat is dissipated by a combination of convection (loss of heat by circulatory transmission of blood) and radiation (heat transmission through radiant energy) with a small portion being lost by vaporization (heat dispelled through perspiration).

When environmental temperature approaches skin temperature (approximately 92° F.) heat loss through convection and radiation gradually comes to an end. When environmental temperatures rise above skin temperatures, the only means for heat loss is evaporation of sweat. Sweating then becomes the only means for the body to lose heat at temperatures above skin temperature. The mere process of sweating is not in itself effective in dissipating heat; liquid sweat must be converted to a gas by evaporation before any heat loss occurs. Sweat that merely rolls off is virtually ineffective, but large heat losses can result when the weather is so dry that the liquid is evaporated from the skin so rapidly that sweating is imperceptible.

When an instructor or participant exercises in a hot and dry environment, cooling of the skin is brought about by evaporation of sweat. No problem from heat cramps, stroke, or exhaustion should occur because air can absorb considerable moisture before becoming saturated. Cooling the skin is not the desired end result of evaporation since the real purpose is to cool the core temperature. Heat is transported from the core to the skin through blood circulation. The volume of the circulatory system increases considerably. Heart rate increases to meet the demand of exercising muscles and skin circulation. Because of these increases to the cardiac system, exercise in temperatures close to or above skin temperature can impose severe loads upon the cardiovascular system, even when the air is relatively dry. Hence, the aerobic instructor must remember that a hot, dry environment is not beneficial to a training effect.

In comparison, evaporative heat loss requires atmospheric conditions that result in evaporation—not dripping of perspiration. When the relative humidity approaches 100, the air is virtually saturated with water vapor and can accept no more from the skin. Perspiration that then drips can have no cooling effect. Without a cooling effect, the body temperature will rise rapidly, until death ensues at 105° to 108° F. Hence while aerobic dancing, it is imperative that environmental temperatures be regulated as to the amount of humidity. We must also remember that with the increased circulatory demands, training effect is diminished. Therefore, the whole purpose of aerobic exercise is useless in a hot, humid environment.

Acceptable Acoustics. An aerobic dance facility must have good acoustic properties. The room has acoustic properties if the aerobic dance music and instructor's voice are properly shaped to reflect useful sound to the participants. The sound cannot have disturbing echoes. A "useful" reflection is one that arrives at the participant within 1/20 of a second after the sound from the instructor and playback device. If the reflection is delayed longer, it becomes a disturbing echo. The materials chosen to muffle sound must control reverberation. Reverberation is a mixture of many small reflected sounds that combine and die away slowly. Reverberations should last no more than one to two seconds if the participants are to hear what is being said. Unfortunately, poor acoustics, besides limiting what the participant can hear, are indirectly harmful for the instructor's voice. If the participants cannot hear because of poor acoustics, the instructor usually yells louder, which results in voice strain or voice injury.

Some possible symptoms of voice strain are: dry throat and mouth (a result of breathing through the mouth accelerated by air-conditioning), frequent clearing of the throat (more than two to three times per hour), cracking voice (using forced, irregular puffs to increase loudness), vocal fatigue (excessive effort), lowered pitch (swelling of or growths on vocals cords), and hoarseness (gravel-like quality).

Adequate Sound Systems.   A quality sound system is an essential ingredient for a successful aerobic dance program. A simple tape deck is ineffective and creates more problems than it's worth for the instructor. An adequate sound system has the following elements:

1. A cordless microphone attachment so the instructor is free to move about. A microphone also helps reduce voice strain.
2. Separate adjustments of the volume and microphone so that the volume on the microphone can be adjusted without affecting the music level.
3. Sound monitors so that the instructors can monitor their own voice loudness as well as the music.
4. Enough speakers to fill the room evenly with sound. If only one speaker is used the sound is too loud at the source and too hard to hear away from the speakers. Also, if the instructor gives commands, more speakers will help the participants hear distinctly.

Such a system is quite expensive, but will save injury to the instructor's voice as well as help all the participants hear clearly.

Clean, Working Showers.   An essential facility for any exercise program is a clean, functional locker room. Participants as well as instructors perspire profusely. After the cool-down, they need a shower to decrease chance of chill. Also, a good warm shower may help decrease fluid buildup in muscles and decrease muscle soreness. One of the current theories to explain muscle soreness during an intense workout is muscle ischemia or lack of blood supply to a muscle. If muscle ischemia is the cause of muscle soreness, a warm shower immediately after exercise will increase the blood supply and may help elevate muscle soreness. Shower facilities will also add an attractive incentive to participants to attend aerobic dance during business lunch hours.

A Bright Cheery Atmosphere.   The participants and instructors will enjoy the aerobic dance experience more if the exercise room is bright, well-lighted, and presents a cheery surrounding. The dance facility lighting must have enough candle power to illuminate the room from one light source to another.

A Final Note About Facilities

Exercise is necessary for all of us, but exercise in poor facilities that places undue risk for injury is not acceptable. Instructors bear an ethical responsibility if they knowingly provide a service in less than adequate facilities, and their participants suffer injury because of those facilities. (For legal ramifications, see Chapter 8).

Equipment

Little equipment outside of an adequate sound system is necessary to provide an aerobic dance program. However, extra amenities will make the participants more comfortable.

Exercise Pads.   Since a good aerobic dance program addresses all the components of health-related fitness, the participant will need an exercise mat or pad. Just about any soft, pliable, foam material will do. However, in order to keep the facility and the participants clean, a mat covered with a cleanable, nonporous surface is best. Numerous commercial mats are available, though most are over priced. Budget stores carry foam padding that will serve as a mat for a relatively inexpensive cost.

Hand or Ankle Weights.   No hand or ankle weights are acceptable in aerobic exercise because of possible joint injury. (See Chapter 7: Aerobic Dance Injuries.)

Progressive Resistance Weights.   Some aerobic dance programs use one-pound to five-pound weights as additional resistance in their strength-building program. The theory is that participants will increase muscle tone, endurance, and definition by doing numerous repetitions. However as you remember from Chater 2, we do not recommend using light weights with numerous repetitions to develop muscle tone and endurance. It is true that numerous repetitions (15 or more) with a light hand or foot weight is beneficial in developing muscle tone, definition, and endurance. Muscle endurance is developed by overloading (60 to 80 percent of maximum) the muscle. That is, if a participant can only do 10 repetitions of a resistance exercise, increasing the number of repetitions will increase muscle endurance. However, serious joint stress can occur with numerous repetitions of any exercise, let alone with the additional one-to five-pound hand or foot weight.

Personal Participant Equipment

Dress.   What to wear to an aerobic dance class is each individual's choice. However, the instructor and participant must remember basic exercise physiology and temperature regulation (see above) in selecting an aerobic dance costume.

1. Wear only cotton material. Cotton breathes and permits evaporation to occur. The body will regulate its temperature better and will have less chance of overheating. The purpose of aerobic exercise is to develop cardiovascular efficiency, not just to sweat.

2. Wear loose-fitting clothing. Loose clothing lets more air to the body and aids the evaporation and cooling process.

3. Stay away from nylon hose, tights, or leotards. They do not breathe and keep the body too warm.

4. In a warm environment, do not wear warm-ups during aerobic conditioning. Many participants want to hide their bodies during exercise so they wear heavy warm-ups. Or they believe that increased sweating will help them lose more weight. It is true that sweating increases water weight loss. However, the weight lost is quickly regained. Fat loss occurs only through oxidation of storage fat.

5. Wear clean, holeless cotton socks. Cotton absorbs moisture. Well fitting, holeless socks will decrease the chance of blisters.

Shoes.   Much research has been done on aerobic dance shoes in the last five years, and the results are important to every instructor and participant. Dance aerobics, high or low impact, is unique in the amount of joint stress placed on the body. Most stress injuries are best managed through modification of training practices, exercise surfaces, or aerobic shoes. However, certain individuals fail to respond to these conservative measures and require modification of the shoe-foot interface. Specifically, these individuals suffer from a combination of the following structural foot variations such as: excess foot pronation, calcaneous valgus or varus (heel turned in and out Figure 4-3), and forefoot valgus or varus.

Typically a worn shoe will show the signs of wear from each type of structural foot abnormality. A foot that remains in pronation too long typically shows extreme wear on the outside heel and inside toe of the shoe. Extreme valgus stress wears the inside of heel. No individual has anatom-

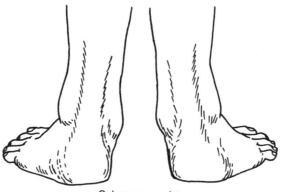

FIGURE 4-3   Calcaneous valgus

ically correct feet, though the body manages most normal levels of exercise stress. Individuals who run, engage in heavy exercise activity, or perform aerobic dance may require a shoe-foot interface to control excess anatomical abnormality.

The shoe-foot interface is commonly called a foot orthotic device. This device maintains the ankle subtaler joint (the joint between the Talus and Calcaneous bones) in a neutral position, and supports the medial longitudinal arch.

The orthotic device is custom fit by a physician, physical therapist, or podiatrist to correct for each foot's anatomical abnormality. A plaster cast is made while the subtaler, talonavicular, and forefoot are in neutral positions. The plaster cast is then sent to an orthotic laboratory for fabrication of the device. Depending on the company, the orthotic device can be designed for participation in just about any type of exercise activity. The device corrects the improper foot alignment as it contacts a surface, thus reducing the stresses encountered in the foot, shin, leg, hip, and lower back.

While most individuals can benefit from some type of orthotic device, the cost is usually prohibitive. The fitting and device costs approximately $300. In addition, the majority of people suffering from lower body stress injuries may still encounter injury even with an orthotic when exercising through repetitive movements such as aerobic dance. The device mainly reduces the potential for greater stress injury. Therefore, we recommend that people who cannot jump rope without pain should avoid an aerobic dance program. In Chapter 7 we discuss shoe construction thoroughly.

A Final Note. Adequate facilities are essential for a succesful aerobic dance program. Flooring space and construction help eliminate numerous injuries. Correct ventilation is imperative if participants are to function effectively in the exercise setting. And a cheery, bright atmosphere with good showers presents an attractive functional facility.

Equipment, other than a functional sound system, is not necessary. Exercise mats add another dimension to the aerobic dance experience but hand weights are not prescribed. A participant's personal equipment should be functional and effective but serve their unique needs.

chapter
5

Skilled as a Teacher

HOW TO DEVELOP AN AEROBIC DANCE

Introduction

An aerobic dance is any exercise utilizing groups of large muscles and performed to music. To choreograph an aerobic dance is not difficult; all that is needed is to hear a beat, count, and follow acceptable training techniques. Of course, some dance background makes choreography much easier. Before choreographing an aerobic dance, whether it be a warm-up, cool-down, high-impact, or low-impact aerobics, take the following factors into consideration:

1. Participants' age and fitness level
2. Participants' dance experience
3. Participants' body balance, alignment, and control

Participants' Age and Fitness Level

Fit, young people enjoy aerobic dance. High-impact aerobics when done three times a week for 20 to 40 minutes is stimulating, invigorating, throughly enjoyable, and develops total fitness. Fit, young people can participate with few injuries and little discomfort.

However, middle-aged, overweight individuals who have done little exercise should not be enrolled in a high-intensity dance aerobic workout. (For pregnant participants see Chapter 9). It would be wise to place such participants and any other nonfit participants in a low-impact aerobics class or a modified calisthenics class. These participants may incur injury and will definitely suffer muscle soreness, joint stress, and overall fatigue, which usually deters them from returning to an exercise program. To provide them with a safe, successful aerobic exercise, develop their aerobic choreography by emphasizing walking and nonlocomotor motions, i.e., swinging, swaying, bending, stretching, twisting, and turning. Use various calisthenic exercises within their routines, such as tummy tucks, shoulder shrugs, and arm circles. Because of their fitness level, they will reach aerobic training effect quickly with what a fit individual would consider little work.

Also because of their poor fitness, these participants need to concentrate on proper body alignment, body control, and kinesthesia. Few of them will be able to follow the instructor's demonstration of correct technique. We recommend that classes for these individuals be kept small, under thirty, and that two instructors be available: one leading and one on the floor watching, helping, correcting, and motivating.

Participants' Dance Experience

Individuals with dance experience love an aerobic class that is choreographed with difficult jazz movements. The trickier the better, and they thrive on new choreography. The choreography becomes a contest between the instructor and participants, with the instructor providing new dances each session. The participants get bored easily and demand freshness, quality, and intricacy.

But the average participant is just the opposite. Difficult jazz movements are beyond their ability. They want choreography that is easy to learn. They want the dances to be repetitive. And they want to be able to learn a routine and know that they will do it again and again.

Participants' Body Balance, Alignment, and Control

Novice dancers, nonathletes, or obese populations may have difficulty maintaining body balance, alignment, and control. As in Figures 5-1 and 5-2, the model is out of alignment and unbalanced. Participants who typically perform while unbalanced and unaligned have more than an average chance of suffering some type of exercise injury. They typically do not (1) keep their center of gravity over their line of gravity; (2) have kinesthetic

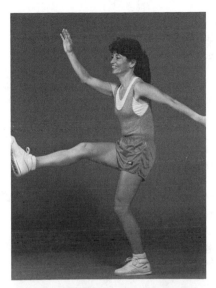

FIGURE 5-1

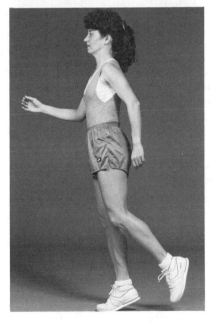

FIGURE 5-2

and body awareness; (3) control their bodily movements; or (4) know how to absorb force.

Center of Gravity. Center of gravity over line of gravity is a basic mechanical law that must be followed while performing any task. Line of gravity is an imaginary gravitational line that flows through the body to the center of the earth. The center of gravity is the earth's gravitational pull on the body. In females, the center of gravity is usually centered low in the body at the hips and thighs. For males, the center of gravity usually is higher, around the shoulders. Because of this center of gravity difference between males and females, each gender is limited in its ability to perform certain tasks. For example, women cannot run as fast or jump as high as men. In contrast, men do not have as much balance as women.

In performing any balanced activity, the body's center of gravity must fall within the line of gravity. When we stand, sit, pose, and so forth, the center of gravity must be in alignment with the earth's line of gravity. If the center of gravity shifts outside the body's line of gravity, balance is lost. Loss of balance is not necessarily wrong because it is essential for our movement patterns. That is, in order to perform any locomotion skills, we must shift the body's center of gravity outside the line of gravity. For instance, walking is a losing and regaining of balance (see Figure 5-3). The body leans forward from the ankle, the center of gravity then shifts forward outside the body's line of gravity. Balance is lost as the body falls forward. Balance is regained when a step is taken. By constantly losing and regaining balance, we are able to walk. However, if the center of gravity shifts too far outside the line of gravity, the body will not be able to regain balance.

If the body is inefficient and awkward in regaining balance, the result is clumsiness. Watch a toddler try to walk and see inefficient mastery of

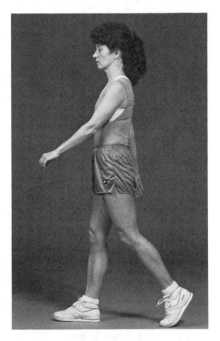

FIGURE 5-3

balance lost and regained. In contrast, watch any great NFL running back. They have the ability to place the center of gravity far outside the line of gravity and still be able to regain their balance. They have learned how to maintain balance even while being hit, twisted, or turned by their opponents.

In aerobic dance, most participants do not have such mechanical skills. They violate the law of center of gravity over line of gravity, with adverse effects. These participants are awkward and clumsy in their locomotor skills. Their center of gravity is often too far forward, backward, or sideward. When the instructor is moving quickly from one step to another, these participants are always moving the wrong way. They lumber through class, can never keep up, and constantly feel like an ostrich in a flock of swans. Other body parts or soft tissues must compensate for the inability to maintain balance, thus increasing the potential for injuries such as ankle, knee, thigh, hip, and low back sprains or strains.

Without thinking, individuals with a good kinesthetic awareness are able to efficiently perform this movement through easy as well as complex patterns. For example, on side-to-side movements, the foot contacts the floor and forces are absorbed by the foot, bent knee, hip, and low back (Figures 5-4, 5-5). The upper body shifts the line of gravity back over the center of gravity and balance is regained.

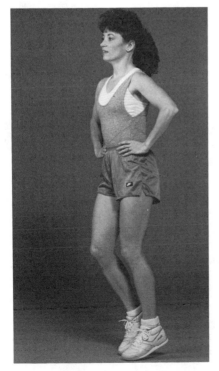

FIGURE 5-4

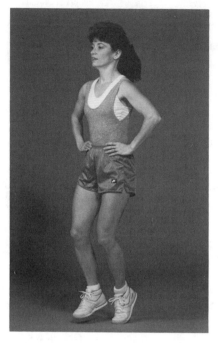

FIGURE 5-5

However, individuals who are overweight, pregnant, or have unde-veloped kinesthtic awareness perform these movements extremely ineffi-ciently. The movement is jerky, and many times they fall or quickly have to shift their opposite foot in the same direction to regain balance. An over-weight or pregnant individual has an increased stress on the low back, knee, hip, and ankle because of the additional weight.

In a normal standing position their center of gravity is shifted outside their body. Therefore, to keep the line of gravity over the center of gravity their back is placed in lumbar lordosis (an abnormal anterior curvature of the spine, or the typical swayback). This curvature places extreme stress on the vertebral discs and surrounding soft tissues. The stress is further aggra-vated by a movement pattern that forces the line of gravity even further outside the body's center of gravity. Typical· of this condition are weak abdominal muscles, tightening of the lower back extensor muscles, and contraction of the lumbar fascia. The result can be lumbar ligamentous spain or muscular strain. Also, the pubic arch lowers in lordosis, which produces a corresponding lift of the ischial tuberosity, where the hamstring muscles attach. Consequently, the potential for hamstring muscle strains increases. In addition, the lumbar and hip regions become extremely inflexible.

Both sprains and strains can easily occur when movements are fast and jerky. Acute injuries such as knee and ankles sprains, muscle strains, and low back injury can typically occur. In addition, these people are concentrating so much on the movement itself that they forget the basic principle of absorption of forces. The jarring jerky movements place further stress on the body's soft tissues, causing further injury potential.

Kinesthetic and Body Awareness. Kinesthetic and body awareness is the body's ability to know where it is: in relation to itself, in relation to space, and in relation to others. Kinesthesia (Kinetics – motion, thesia – awareness) or movement awareness is information from specific internal body receptors or proprioceptors located in the skin, joints, muscles, and semicircular canals, that informs us about our current status. Kinesthesia tells us, without using our special sensory receptors of eyes, ears, and nose, where our arms are; are they bent at the elbow or wrist? Are they hanging at our sides or stretching over our heads? Kinesthesia tells us where our trunk is in relation to our limbs. Are we sitting down or standing up? Kinesthesia tells us where we are in relation to the space around us? Are we turning, twisting, swinging, swaying, or standing motionless?

A dancer, gymnast, or any athlete has a keen kinesthetic awareness. They know where their bodily parts are at all times. However, the average aerobic dance participant has not developed this kinesthetic ability. They have little concept of where their arms and legs are in relation to their trunks. These participants randomly move their body parts. They have no concept of degrees or levels of motion. Because of their poor kinesthetic sense, they have great difficulty in following or mimicking the instructor.

Body awareness is the ability to know where one is in space as well as in relation to others. Body awareness is knowing how close the participants beside, in front, and behind are. Body awareness is imperative to making sure that the participants do not collide.

Body Control. Body control is being able to have keen kinesthetic awareness combined with body awareness and following the laws of physics. Body control is also having the ability to change any motion at any given time. Body control is preventing the body from doing free-flowing activities, i.e., activities that the participant cannot control. Many participants violate the body control principle as they forcefully and deliberately move a body part. They produce too much force through acceleration of muscle contraction times the mass of their body parts. The result is stress on joints, ligamentous, and tendonous tissue.

Absorption of Force. Force absorption is the force that is assumed by an object or a person. We can efficiently reduce force assumed by our bodies by increasing the surface area and the distance or time over which force is received. In aerobic dance, this basic mechanical principle is very important, because inefficient force absorption is the main culprit in stress injury.

Placed in perspective, this means that as participants move, they must

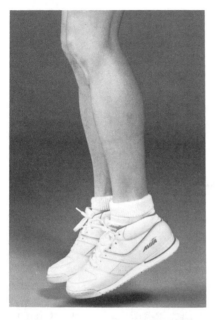

FIGURE 5-6

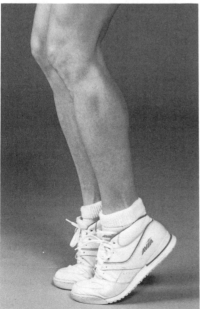

FIGURE 5-7

somehow apply the principle of increased surface area on landing and increased time or distance. Mechanically, the human body can only absorb force by use of joint absorption. By giving and bending through a series of joints, force is absorbed. Figures 5-6, 5-7, 5-8, and 5-9 show a sequence of

FIGURE 5-8

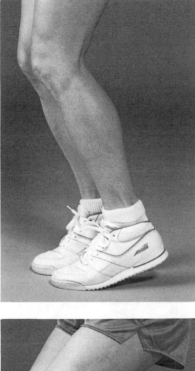

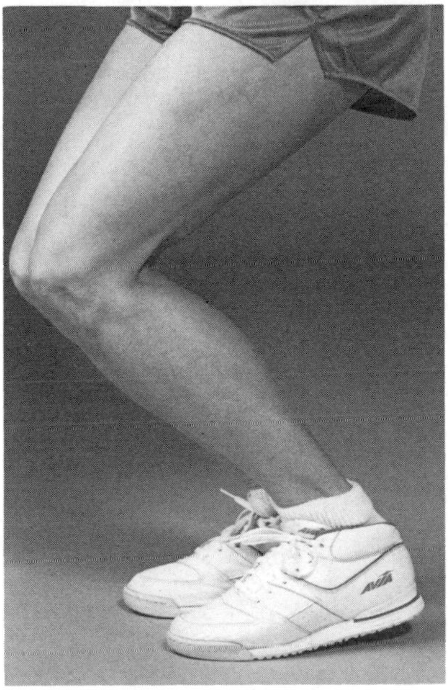

FIGURE 5-9

absorbing force for surface and distance. In Figure 5-6, the body is air-
borne and about to land—notice that the toes are reaching for the surface.
In Figure 5-7, the toes have made contact, are bent and absorbing force. In
Figures 5-8 and 5-9 the ankles, knees, hips, and even the vertebrae have
bent to absorb the force. By bending and giving, the force has been
absorbed over time and distance. The time and distance is the bending all
sequential joints.

   How to Teach Body Alignment, Kinesthesia, and Body Control.   To learn
body alignment, kinesthetic awareness, and body control requires much
time and effort by the participant. As an instructor, incorporate specific
exercises into the program that will increase these abilities for the participants. However, to learn body alignment, kinesthesia, and body control
requires practice both outside, as well as, in-class work. As in learning any
new skill, the body requires practice in order to make the movement patterns and abilities second nature.
   Typically, people who have sustained an injury to the ankle, knee,
hip, or low back regions will experience poor balance abilities with that
body segment. They may perform well on the uninjured side, but because
of the injury proprioceptors on the injured side need to be retrained. They
must relearn proprioceptive awareness.
   Improving kinesthetic awareness involves teaching the body's internal
receptors to understand where the body or segment is in time and space.
Specifically, the body's proprioceptors, located in the golgi tendon bodies,
must determine degrees of joint angles, limb, and body movements. The
proprioceptors (sensory receptors located in joints, muscles, and the inner
ear) come into play when joints try to maintain an upright posture through
abnormal unbalanced movements. For instance, individuals who continually sprain ankles may have underdeveloped proprioceptive awareness.
Rather than the proprioceptors activating the muscles to contract on the
opposite side of the stress, balance is lost and a sprain may occur.
   We all practiced kinesthetic awareness as children. Stand with the
arms to the side, close your eyes, and attempt to keep balance. This task
require proprioceptors to work. Specifically, as the body starts to lose balance proprioceptors on the opposite side from the balance loss are acti-
vated. This keeps the body in an upright, balanced position.
   Balance becomes more difficult as we perform the same task on one
foot. Open the eyes, raise one leg behind the body, and place the arms
perpendicular to the body. The proprioceptors are constantly activating to
maintain balance. In addition, the eyes are extremely important for maintaining balance. The eyes focus on objects to help the body maintain an
upright and balanced posture. Perform the above task with the eyes closed
and feel how difficult retaining balance becomes. Any task that requires the

body to balance on one foot with the arms to the side of the body requires more effort to balance.

Therefore any variation of the above activities will increase proprioception abilities. These can easily be incorporated into the warm-up and cool-down program phase. The proprioceptor work can be the transition phases between one flexibility or stretching task and another.

Learning body control requires plenty of space to move unimpeded. Beginners must take smaller steps compared to the advanced individuals. By taking smaller steps, the line of gravity falls closer to the body's center of gravity. Have these individuals count an extra beat while in contact with the floor. This means the participant will spend more time in contact with the floor surface, reduce potential microtrauma, and increase balance, body awareness, and body control.

Watch the participants closely; you will notice that many do not perform controlled arm or leg movements. The degree to which they move their arms and legs does not match yours. Typically, they are concentrating so much on staying with the beat and moving in the same direction that they move segments quickly and in an uncontrolled way.

An easy method to teach arm control is to have an eight-count beat. The advanced people could move their arms to an overhead position on four counts then down to finish the eight-count sequence. The beginners would perform the overhead arm up movement once to an eight-count beat and down to eight-counts. Through the addition of extra counts for the beginners there is less movement between each count. Therefore they should gain a better controlled movement pattern.

The difficulty arises in having the participants perform the same movement to different counts. A remedy would be to have one of the better participants stand in the front of the room to lead the advanced people, as the instructor leads the beginners through their counting sequence. As the beginners learn the controlled movements they can then shorten the count to four beats. All aerobic dance movement can incorporate this principle. Be creative and add kinesthetic awareness activities and controlled movement patterns to your program.

Teaching Force Absorption. In order to teach force absorption, slow down the actions and have the participants feel the action as joints bend and give with the force. For example, practice a jump without leaving the ground. The participant can learn force absorption through the full range, from toes, ankles, hips, to vertebrae (Figures 5-10, 5-11, 5-12). Practice slowly without leaving the ground. Do this several times. Then add a short jump, and absorb force through each joint. With practice, participants will learn the feel of absorbing force through all the joints. This same technique can be used for hops, leaps, running, and so forth.

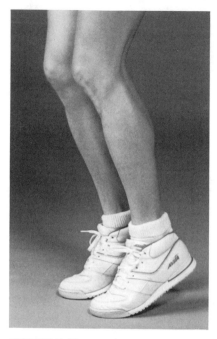

FIGURE 5-10

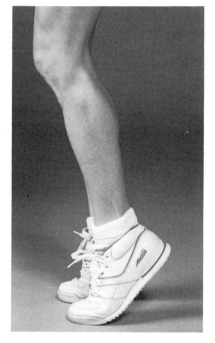

FIGURE 5-11

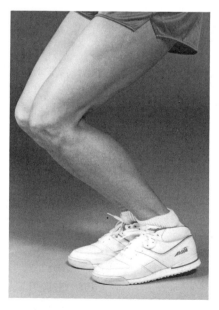

FIGURE 5-12

CHOREOGRAPHY FOR AN AEROBIC DANCE

After taking into account the participant's fitness level, age, dance experience, body alignment, kinesthesia, and body control, we can begin our choreography process.

To choreograph a warm-up, cool-down, high-impact or low-impact routine for the average, fit participant follow these eight cardinal rules.

EIGHT CARDINAL RULES OF AEROBIC DANCE CHOREOGRAPHY

1. Choose lyricless music. Lyrics tend to drown out the instructor's cues.
2. Choose music that fits the audience. Middle-aged individuals like the oldies sound. Young people like current rock.
3. Select music to match your fitness intent. For high-impact or low-impact aerobics, choose music with a moderate to fast beat, about 100 to 120 beats per minute for high-impact and low-impact aerobics. Too fast or too slow a beat is hard to follow and perform. Select a slow tempo for the warm-up and cool-down.
4. Listen to the music and think of what movements might fit its style.
5. Count out all the measures and determine where the music repeats itself by verses and chorus.
6. Select a movement that fits each verse or chorus.
7. Keep the movement pattern the same up to a maximum of 32 counts then change to a different movement. Doing one movement more than 32 counts tends to cause muscle fatigue as well as place stress on a joint.
8. Keep the patterns simple.

Incorporating the Locomotor and Nonlocomotor Skills

Before we begin, we should review the elements that are available to us as choreographers. Basically, all that is available are the simple locomotor and nonlocomotor movements. The locomotor skills are: walk, run, jump, hop, leap, skip, gallop, and slide. The nonlocomotor skills are: twist-turn, bend-stretch, swing-sway, and push-pull.

The Locomotor Skills

Walk. Walking is a movement of the body in a forward direction by transferring weight from one foot to another with a heel, to ball of foot, to toe action. The arms swing in opposition (see Figure 5-13).

Walking is the simplest and probably most efficient form of locomotion that we may engage in, probably because of the developmental pattern of the individual and his practice and proficiency in it over the years.

The position of the body is similar to that for standing, except that the center of gravity is moved forward so that inertia may be overcome and force applied to move the body in the desired direction. The act of walking is a matter of disturbing the mechanical equilibrium of the body and form-

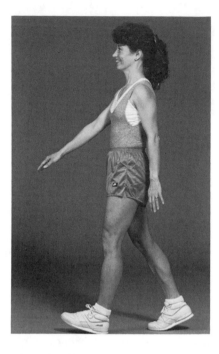

FIGURE 5-13

ing successive new bases by moving the legs forward alternately. Because the body moves forward as a unit, walking may be described as a linear movement caused by the rotary movement of the legs. When the weight is moved forward, the foot acts as an axis and the upper end of the leg moves forward about it. This is followed by swinging the foot forward and the establishment of a new base. During this movement the upper part of the leg moves about the axis of the hip.

In analyzing the walk we find that each leg goes through two separate phases, the swinging phase and the supporting phase.

The swinging phase begins as soon as the leg has exerted its backward push against the ground. The first action is flexing at the hip joint, followed by a flexing of the knee and ankle. The flexion of the ankle returns the foot from the extended position it assumed while pushing against the ground to its normal alignment with the leg. As the leg begins to move under the body, the flexion of each of the joints becomes more pronounced. The swinging motion is begun by muscular contraction of the hip, but is aided by gravity and momentum. As the foot clears the ground, the knee begins to extend, and the foot is brought back into position to contact the ground again.

The heel is the first part of the foot to strike the ground because the ankle is flexed. The striking of the heel on the ground is the distinguishing feature of walking, and is usually emphasized in teaching children to walk. As the heel strikes the ground, the weight is spread along the foot, heel, outer side of the foot, and toes, where the push for the next step is applied. The rolling movement of the foot from heel to toe cushions the shock of impact with the ground and provides a gradual absorption of force.

During each step there is a time when both feet are in contact with the ground. As the weight shifts onto the ball of the leading foot, the heel of the trailing foot will strike the ground and most of the body weight will be shifted to it. The more slowly we walk, the more the overlap in the supportive phases of the two feet.

As in any form of motion, inertia must be overcome by the force of the foot pushing against the ground and by the pull of gravity as the weight of the body is transferred forward.

Just before stepping forward, the trunk is inclined toward the direction in which we will be walking. This forward leaning of the trunk is used to place the center of gravity in line with the force exerted by the driving leg. Walking has been described as a process of pushing the body off balance and then regaining balance with the supportive leg. Speed of walking is accelerated by increasing the angle of forward lean and length of stride.

Run. A run is a movement similar to the walk. However, there is a period of nonsupport where the weight of the body is not touching the floor (Figures 5-14, 5-15, 5-16, 5-17). The weight is taken on the ball of the foot. The arms swing in opposition.

FIGURE 5-14

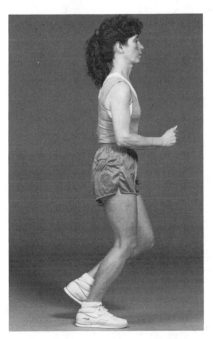

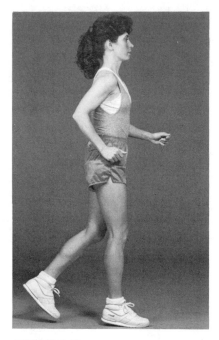

FIGURE 5-15

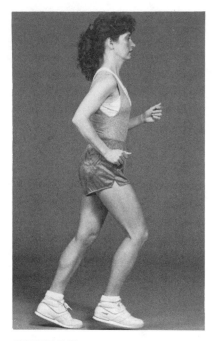

FIGURE 5-16

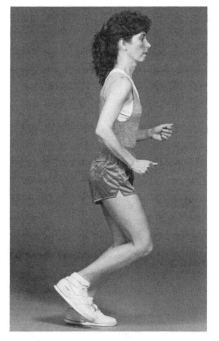

FIGURE 5-17

The principles of body mechanics for running are quite similar to those in walking, particularly the opposed movement of arms and legs. The primary difference is the reduction or elimination of the supportive phase. The time to change from a walk to a run is about when the speed of locomotion exceeds 4 mph. A running gait becomes less fatiguing than the forced rate of walking, although the energy consumption is increased.

In running, as in walking, swinging of the arms and legs must be coordinated in order to balance the rotatory effect of the leg swing on the trunk. The swing of the arms is much more vigorous in the run, and the elbow is invariably bent in order to allow rapid movement with as little effort as possible (Figure 5-18). With the elbow always flexed during the arm swing, the tendency to swing the arms across the body is emphasized. As speed is increased, the swing should be less diagonal so that the force can be more directly backward and forward. A runner with heavy hips and legs in relation to her arms and shoulders must carry the arms farther from the body or increase the vigor of the arm swing to balance the force of her legs.

All movements should be in the direction of the run in order not to detract from the efficiency of movement. Knees should be moved as much in a straight line as possible and should be as straight as possible, only inward enough to counterbalance the rotation of the hips (Figure 5-19).

The efficiency of the run can be increased by emphasis on lifting the knee forward, relaxing the shoulders, and bending the elbows so that the arms can swing in a natural position. When the arm is bent at the elbow in a

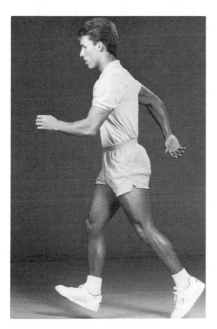

FIGURE 5-18

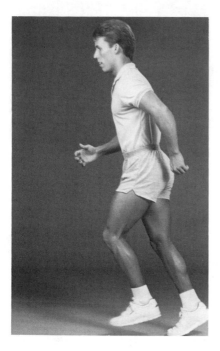

FIGURE 5-19

natural position, with the lower arm diagonally in front of the body, the arms will hold themselves away from the body in the desired position. An outward rotation will tend to push the arms against the trunk. Exercises which relax the shoulder girdle and upper arm and move the arms independently of the trunk will be helpful. Some authors have suggested holding the thumb against the tip of the second or third finger (instead of making a fist) to prevent tension in the arm muscles. The muscles used to press the thumb against one of these fingers are located in the forearm, while clenching the fist involves muscles of the entire arm, and thus may cause tensions which will restrict arm action.

Because of the angle of the femur caused by a wider pelvis, women may have some mechanical disadvantage in running. Some suggestions follow for increasing the running efficiency of women: (1) the knee should be lifted more (2) the upper arms should be permitted to swing more freely and the lower arms should be kept closer to the body, and (3) the knees should be bent and carried straight forward in order to reduce lateral sway (Figure 5-20).

In aerobic dance, choreography often is designed to run in an arc. To overcome the tendency of a moving body to continue in a straight line, it is necessary to apply force toward the outside of the arc by leaning the body in toward the center of the circle. The inward lean of the body will cause the force of the leg drive to be outward in addition to downward and backward, and the pressure on the surface will move the body inward as well as forward. Because of the diagonal force applied while running in a circle, friction is important to prevent slipping.

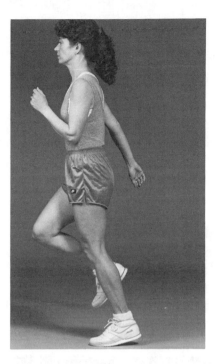

FIGURE 5-20

Jump.   A jump is a take-off from one or both feet and a landing on both feet. The arms move in parallel and upward or forward direction (Figures 5-21, 5-22, 5-23).

FIGURE 5-21

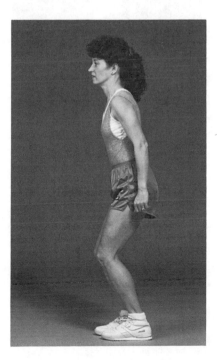

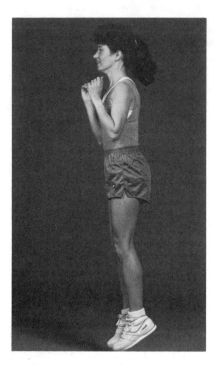

FIGURE 5-22

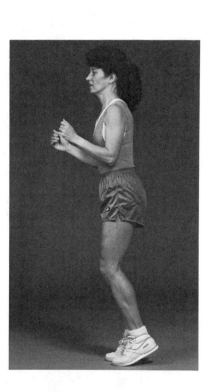

FIGURE 5-23

Hop.   A hop is a take-off from one foot with a landing on the same foot. Movement is produced by pushing action of the foot and the simultaneous parallel and upward lift of the arms (Figures 5-24, 5-25).

FIGURE 5-24

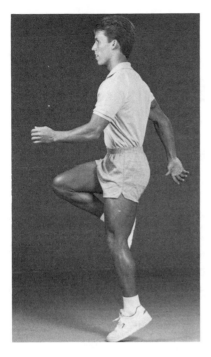

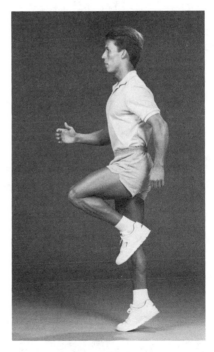

FIGURE 5-25

Leap.   A leap is an extension of the body in an upward and forward direction. The take-off is from one foot and the landing is on the other. The leap is an extended run (Figures 5-26, 5-27, 5-28).

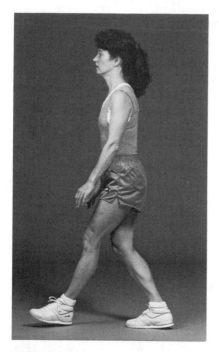

FIGURE 5-26

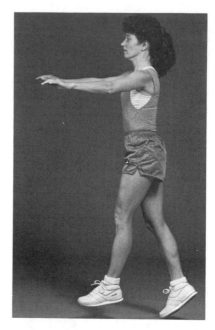

FIGURE 5-27

FIGURE 5-28

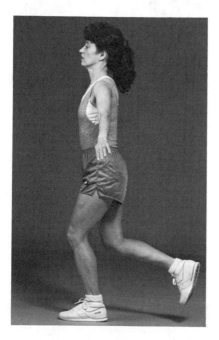

Jumping, leaping, and hopping are all forms of movement where the body is projected through the air by the propulsive force of the legs. The physical laws which govern any projectile apply to the flight of the body.

When the projecting force is exerted by either one foot or both feet, and the landing is made by both feet striking the ground at the same time, the movement is defined as a jump. If the propulsive force is exerted by one foot and the landing made on the other foot, the movement is defined as a leap. If the propulsive force is exerted by one foot and the landing made on the same foot, the movement is defined as a hop.

There are many different types of jumps, hops, and leaps which have many varied applications such as side-to-side jumps, (Figure 5-29), step hop, step kick (Figure 5-30), and pony steps (Figures 5-31, 5-32).

FIGURE 5-29

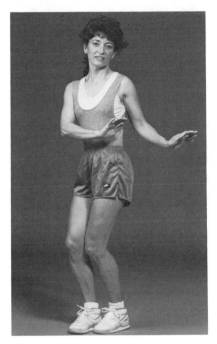

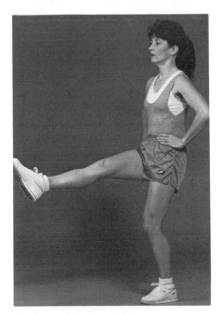

FIGURE 5-30

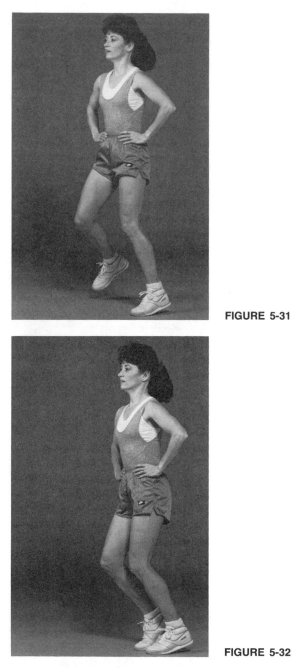

FIGURE 5-31

FIGURE 5-32

Skip.   A skip is a step and a hop on alternating feet with arms swing-ing in opposition. The skill is performed to an uneven rhythm pattern (Figure 5-33).

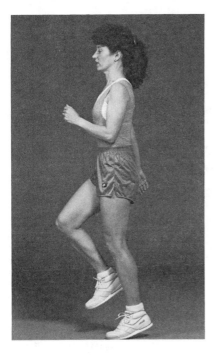

FIGURE 5-33

The skipping action puts two fundamental movement patterns, the step and the hop, together into a combined pattern of movement. There is a three-stage developmental sequence which serves as the basis for the following description. The skip is a continuous flow of the step and the hop involving rhythmical alternation of the leading foot. A skip is a rhythmical weight transfer throughout the movement. A rhythmical use of the arms aids momentum during the time of the weight transfer. There is a low vertical lift on the hop phase of the skip and the landing is on the toe or ball of the foot.

Gallop and Slide. The gallop is a step, leap, step. As one foot leaps forward, weight is changed to the opposite leg. The leading leg then steps. A good leap shows mastery of lean forward, arms swinging freely at shoulder, heel-toe foot action of lead foot, and momentary suspension in air. Variations including the backward gallop or side slide.

Nonlocomotor Skills

Bend and Stretch. A bend is an action which brings body parts closer together, while a stretch moves body parts further from each other (Figure 5-34). The more technical terms for bend and stretch are flexion and extension.

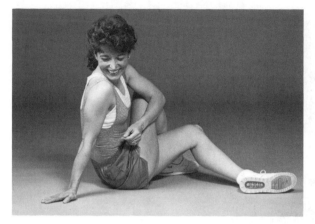

FIGURE 5-34

Twist and Turn.   A twist is the rotation of the body or body part around its longitudal axis. The trunk of the body can be twisted or rotated around the spinal column. In a trunk twist the feet remain stationary while the trunk is rotated to face in different directions. In a twist one point of the axis remains fixed or stationary. The arm can be twisted so that the palm of the hand faces in different directions. The point of the axis at the shoulder remains fixed. The trunk and arms lend themselves best to twisting. Other body parts can be twisted. However, the ease and amplitude of the rotation is limited by body structure (Figure 5-35).

A turn is accomplished by describing a circular air pattern in space. The total body is turned in space by allowing the feet to pivot or step around to face the same direction as the front of the body. Body parts or limbs also can describe circular air patterns. Like the bend and stretch, the twist and turn is experienced first in isolation and then progresses to expressive movement and finally movement with accompaniment.

Push and Pull.   A push is an action in which movement and force is directed away from the center of the body outward. The pull involves force directed inward toward the body. Thus, a push would send an object away from the body while a pull brings objects toward the body.

Swing and Sway.   The main difference between a swing and a sway is the location of the fixed point and the resulting movement in relation to this point. In a swing the fixed point is located about the movement while gravity aids the movement in a pendular fashion. The arm can swing from a fixed point being the shoulder, or swing the leg from the hip or even the upper trunk while bent forward from the waist or the hips. A swaying action involves the base of support as the fixed point while movement occurs above this point by leaning in various directions. The larger the base of support the greater the magnitude of the sway; for example, a larger

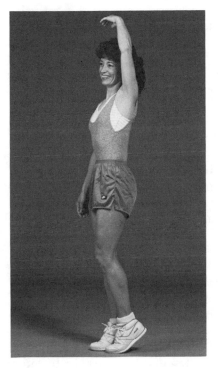

FIGURE 5-35

base of support allows a greater range of movement above the base before the line of gravity falls outside the base than does a smaller base of support. Most commonly, swaying occurs over the feet as the base of support; however, other body parts could be the base of support while swaying occurs over the base.

Using the Locomotor and Nonlocomotor Skills in Choreography

All choreography uses these skills to develop dances, routines, and so forth. If we consider these skills, plus our Eight Cardinal Rules, we can develop an aerobic dance.

To give you an idea of how this works, we chose a fast-paced fifties song by the Big Bopper, "Chantilly Lace." Our intent is high-impact aerobics for a group of fit, experienced, earlier middle-aged participants. We first listened to the music and decided that we could include variations of three simple locomotor skills.

1. Running forward, running backward, running sideward.
2. Jumps with simultaneous claps.
3. Charleston Step (a step, kick, step, step)
4. Step forward and step back with simultaneous finger clicks.

We then counted out the music by measure, counting 1,2 for each measure. We placed the measures in order by verses and choruses (Table 5-1).

This song is quite simple; it has three verses and three choruses. Hence, when we choreograph we find a pattern that will repeat for the verses and the choruses. We may change the pattern for each verse if we want; we chose not to.

(Most fast music has eight measures to a phrase with two beats to a measure. That is a total of 16 counts to a phrase. We usually change the movement pattern after 16 counts.)

We then place our locomotor skills into a pattern within each musical phrase. For "Chantilly Lace," we choreographed the following (Table 5-2).

Most music can be choreographed using the same simple technique. For high-impact aerobics, the variations are limitless since eight locomotor skills, walking, running, hopping, skipping, leaping, galloping, sliding, and jumping, plus the nonlocomotor skills of swinging, swaying, turning, twisting, stretching, and bending can be used. In high impact, increase intensity by including some variation of a controlled arm motion simultaneously with the locomotor skills. We recommend that gastrocemius, anterior tibialis, and hamstring stretching be included within high-impact aerobic choreography. A good stretch will decrease lactic acid build-up during aerobic routines If the choreography is high impact, with variations of hops, participants may have a burning sensation in the calves. The burning is a build-up of lactic acid. The best way to eliminate lactic acid is to chore-

TABLE 5-1. Counting and Choreography.

"Chantilly Lace," Big Bopper; Music begins with a ringing bell, and "Hello, baby," begin counting:

Counts
1-2
2-2
3-2
4-2   Phrase one, Verse one
5-2
6-2
7-2
8-2

1-2
2-2
3-2
4-2   Phrase two, Verse one
5-2
6-2
7-2
8-2

TABLE 5-1 (continued)

1-2	
2-2	
3-2	
4-2	Phrase three, Verse one
5-2	
6-2	
7-2	
8-2	
1-2	
2-2	
3-2	
4-2	Phrase four, Verse one
5-2	
6-2	
7-2	
8-2	
1-2	
2-2	
3-2	
4-2	Phrase one, Chorus
5-2	
6-2	
7-2	
8-2	
1-2	
2-2	
3-2	
4-2	Phrase two, Chorus
5-2	
6-2	
7-2	
8-2	
1-2	
2-2	
3-2	
4-2	Phrase three, Chorus
5-2	
6-2	
7-2	
8-2	
1-2	
2-2	
3-2	
4-2	Phrase four, Chorus
5-2	
6-2	
7-2	
8-2	

TABLE 5-2 "Chantilly Lace".

Participants form a large circle, all face in line of direction (counterclockwise) in circle.

Ringing of bell, Hello-baby, (Begin counting)

Phrase One, Verse One

Counts	
1-2	run forward, left and right
2-2	run forward, left and right
3-2	run forward, left and right
4-2	run forward, left and right
5-2	jump ¼ turn to right clap simultaneously
6-2	jump ¼ turn to right clap simultaneously
7-2	jump ¼ turn to right clap simultaneously
8-2	jump ¼ turn to right clap simultaneously

Phrase Two, Verse One

1-2	run backward, left and right
2-2	run backward, left and right
3-2	run backward, left and right
4-2	run backward, left and right
5-2	jump ¼ turn to right clap simultaneously
6-2	jump ¼ turn to right clap simultaneously
7-2	jump ¼ turn to right clap simultaneously
8-2	jump ¼ turn to right clap simultaneously

Phrase Three, Verse One (Face into circle)

1-2	run right sideward, right and left (Do no cross feet)
2-2	run sideward, right and left
3-2	run sideward, right and left
4-2	run sideward, right and left
5-2	jump ¼ turn to right clap simultaneously
6-2	jump ¼ turn to right clap simultaneously
7-2	jump ¼ turn to right clap simultaneously
8-2	jump ¼ turn to right clap simultaneously

Phrase Four, Verse One

1-2	run left sideward, left and right (Do no cross feet)
2-2	run left sideward, left and right
3-2	run left sideward, left and right
4-2	run left sideward, left and right
5-2	jump ¼ turn to right clap simultaneously
6-2	jump ¼ turn to right clap simultaneously
7-2	jump ¼ turn to right clap simultaneously
8-2	jump ¼ turn to right clap simultaneously

Phrase Three, Chorus (Face into circle)

1-2	Step forward right, slide left forward, Clap count one.
2-2	Step forward left, slide right forward, Clap count one.

TABLE 5-2 (continued)

3-2	Step forward right, slide left forward, Clap count one.
4-2	Step forward left, slide right forward, Clap count one.
5-2	Run forward, right, left
6-2	Run forward, right, left
7-2	Run forward, right, left
8-2	Run forward, right, left
	Phrase Four, Chorus
1-2	Step backward right, slide left forward, Clap count one.
2-2	Step backward left, slide right forward, Clap count one.
3-2	Step backward right, slide left forward, Clap count one.
4-2	Step backward left, slide right forward, Clap count one.
5-2	Run backward, right, left
6-2	Run backward, right, left
7-2	Run backward, right, left
8-2	Run backward, right, left

Face in line of direction, and repeat verse 1 and chorus, three times.

ograph a 10 to 15 second stretch break about three times during the 20 minute aerobic dance workout. Examples for these stretches include: achilles tendon stretch, anterior leg stretch, the sprinter's stretch, and hip and thigh stretch (see Table 5-3).

Choreography for the Cool-Down

If the purpose is a warm-up or cool-down, follow the Eight Cardinal Rules plus remember the purpose of the warm-up and cool-down. A warm-up is to prepare the cardiovascular system as well as the major muscle groups for an aerobic workout. A warm-up should begin with a cardiovascular warmup that includes some light locomotor skill such as stepping, walking, slow skips, gallops, or slides. A warm-up should progress to a full body stretching routine. Examples are cited above and in Chapter 2. In selecting warm-up music, choose songs that are peppy but moderately slow. A cool-down is the opposite of a warm-up in bringing the body back to homeostasis. Hence, the choreography is somewhat in reverse: stretching followed by slow locomotor skills. However, the stretching should not begin immediately after an intense aerobic dance. Prepare the participant for the cool-down by selecting slower tempo music for the end of the aerobic dance session. Then move into the stretching phrase and aerobic cool-down.

TABLE 5-3   Stretches for Choreography.

1. Achilles tendon stretch: Extend one leg back in a lunge position. Keep the heels flat on the floor, toes pointing straight ahead, back leg straight, and bend the front knee. The stretch should be felt in the posterior part of the back leg. Perform the same task with the back leg bent to stretch the solius muscle. Repeat with both legs.

2. Anterior leg stretch: stand with the toes on the right foot pointed down and the foot behind approximately one to two feet. Push the anterior aspect of the foot to the ground. The stretch should be felt on the top of the foot (Figure 5-36).

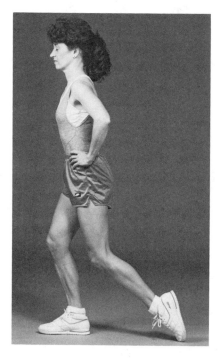

FIGURE 5-36

3. Sprinter's leg stretch: Assume a sprinter's position with one knee bent under the chest, the opposite leg stretched out behind with the heels flat on the floor. The stretch should be felt along the gastrocnemious and hamstring muscles (Figure 5-37).

FIGURE 5-37

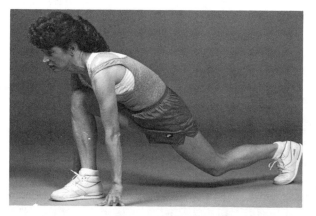

TABLE 5-3   (continued)

4. Hip and thigh stretch: Lean forward with fingers on the ground, the right knee bent under the chest, and left leg extended behind. The bent knee should be directly over its ankle. Lower the hips and feel the stretch on the left thigh and hip (Figure 5-38).

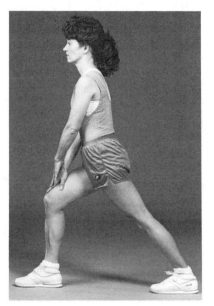

FIGURE 5-38

If the intent is to choreograph for low-impact aerobics, the same rules apply, except the locomotion skills are limited to those in which one foot is always in contact with the floor. The choreography can still be very much like that of high-impact aerobics. Some authorities state that in order to increase intensity for low-impact aerobics, more body parts should be incorporated. However, remember to keep the body in control and limit the number of repetitions. Examples of low-impact aerobic choreography are: Slides, lunges, leg-ups, grapevines, walking, stepping, stepping variations, and so forth.

A Final Note

Choreography can be fun. Participants will enjoy each new routine as long as the choreographer follows the Eight Cardinal Rules and remembers their needs.

6

Skilled
as a Teacher:
Part II

TEACHING TIPS AND TECHNIQUES

Introduction

Many good authorities have written exceptional texts about the art
and science of teaching, and we realize that a few chapters in one text does
not compare with their work. However, a few comments, tips, and techniques may help your teaching.

In general, a good aerobic dance teacher is competent and effective
while motivating and inspiring. We know that students learn best from
teachers who are organized, enthusiastic, competent, and personable. The
best teaching style is relative because no specific teaching style is best.
Students can and do learn from various teaching styles. Whatever style is
chosen, remember student learning comes from teachers who have direction, knowledge, experience, and just the right amount of personality.
Below are some tips and techniques that we use to help students learn.

Teaching Tips

1. Plan Ahead. Organize what is to be taught for a five- to six-week
.period (the time period is arbitrary, it could be two or eight weeks). What is
the long-term goal for each class? When setting this goal know the class's

present fitness level and their present cognitive fitness knowledges. If they are true beginners, set the goals low. Realize that they know little and must begin a learning process. In order to learn anything, whether it is a skill or verbal knowledge, the participant must practice. Plan the teaching to reinforce (letting your participants practice) what they are to learn. If the participants are more advanced, take this into consideration when making your plan. They will be able to progress faster both in their cognitive and skill levels.

2. Be Organized.   Once the long-term goals are planned, organize a daily plan. If you need to make notes to follow, do so. Decide what the class organization is going to be and try to stay on schedule. Don't be creative in changing what's going to happen in class. Participants want constancy in their classes. People are habitual. They like patterns and feel at ease when the class follows the same organizational pattern each time. Get to class early. Have all tapes, tape deck, notes, exercise mats, and whatever other materials are needed. Be organized. Have the tapes ready to play. Don't preview tapes while participants are waiting. Don't have numerous songs on the same tape, unless they are in the order you plan to follow in class. That is, warm-up tapes are followed by calisthenics, followed by aerobic music, and so on. For the participant, there is nothing worse than to get to class and find an instructor who can't find her tapes or is constantly *previewing* to find the right tape.

3. Find a Teaching Style.   There is no best way to teach. In fact, there are numerous ways to teach, such as command style, reciprocal, guided discovery, problem solving, and so forth. None is really better than another. The best teaching style is one in which the instructor is comfortable, relaxed, and at-ease when teaching. Personality is what makes each instructor unique. Use that uniqueness as an asset when teaching. If you do not like people, do not become an aerobic dance instructor.

4. Realize Your Limitations.   Do not be a know-it-all! Students are turned off by instructors who have all the answers. Of course you must be competent, but show a little modesty. Participants see you as an authority, but do not let it go to your head. Realize your limitations and those of your participants.

5. Be a Good Listener.   Most teachers give plenty of instruction and advice. However, a good teacher also listens. A good teacher hears what the participants say through vocal and body language. You can learn much about your teaching by listening for any grumbling or watching for unenthusiastic body action. Take what you hear and see, and improve your teaching. For example, many students will complain at one time or another about some aspect of the class. The difference between a good teacher and a poor teacher is that the good teacher is not offended by the complaints. Listen to what the complaint is, evaluate its meaning, and make a change in your teaching. On the other hand, if you think that what you are teaching is correct and the complaint is unfounded, do not be defensive. Sit down with the students and talk through the problem.

6. Be Personable.   Get to know the students and take an interest in who they are. The more they get to know you, the more motivated they will be to improve. If they see that you care about them, they will work hard.

7. Show a Sense of Humor and Have Fun.   If you enjoy what you teach, your students will probably also. Do not be a task master! Students must understand that exercise is not competition. Encourage your students to enjoy exercise so much that they want to exercise for the rest of their lives. Be supportive: If you approach teaching as a drudgery, the students will know how you feel. Be enthusiastic and fun, and everyone will want to enroll in your class.

Teaching Techniques

Below are listed the pros and cons for a few basic techniques that an aerobic dance instructor may need to communicate and teach an exercise class.

Cueing.   Cueing is verbally prompting or bodily signaling participants to the next choreographed step in the music. Some instructors believe that cueing is a very important aspect of teaching dance exercise. As such, the cue should be brief and called on the preceding measure. Participants will then have enough time to make smooth transitions. Some authorities have described five different verbal cues:

1. Footwork cueing signals each foot to move, right or left.
2. Directional cueing gives the direction to move, such as sideways or forward.
3. Rhythmic cueing gives the correct rhythm of the routine, such as quick (one count), quick, slow (two counts).
4. Numerical cueing counts the rhythm, such as 1, 2, 3, 4.
5. Step cueing gives the name of the step, such as step, hop, step, kick.

As the participants become proficient, they require fewer verbal cues.

However, even though many aerobic dance specialists believe that cueing is important, we question its merit, especially considering scientific data concerning visual and auditory learning. Research shows that auditory cues are delayed. By the time the cue reaches the brain's motor cortex, and is translated, and impulses sent to the muscles to react, the music has passed. This delay may explain why participants have trouble picking up the cue.

Another problem with cueing is the concentration level of the partici-pant. Most beginning to intermediate participants are so busy concentrat-ing on the immediate step, they cannot process a cue to make the transition. Because the human brain cannot process two stimuli at the same time, when the cue is given, the participants typically pause, stumble, or lose the beat. Instructors usually react to the loss of cue by yelling louder, which does not help the participant pick up the cue faster. Yelling louder only causes the instructor voice strain.

Verbal cues are difficult for participants to hear. No matter how low the music, the participants must concentrate to hear the cue. Only the most practiced participant will be able to hear the cue over their own con-centration on the immediate step.

Verbal cues also cause undue voice strain for the instructor. Even with a microphone and the proper sound system, the instructor will place undue strain on the vocal chords to call out the cues.

A final reason to limit verbal cues comes from early research about the function of the right and left brain hemispheres. It was believed that the two hemispheric brains process specific information differently. That is, the right brain supposedly processes all visual, emotional, or abstract information, whereas the left brain is the analytical, factual, verbal process-ing center. Because dance is a visual activity, it would seem logical to teach to the visual or right side of the brain. Hence, some dance researchers believe that learning dance steps is typically a right brain activity. To increase learning, a teacher should reduce or eliminate information to the left half by using few verbal cues or commands. All cues and demonstra-tions should be visual.

We believe that verbal cues should be limited because of voice strain. Visual cues place little or no strain on the voice and are easier for the participants to follow. By keeping the aerobic dance patterns simple and to a constant 16 to 32 beats, the participant can learn to anticipate a change. Also, if the steps are similar or kept to a specific pattern such as always going forward, backward, right sideways, left sideways, or always begin-ning with the same foot, participants can visually pick up cues.

Burnout.   One of the classic problems of working with exercise or service populations is instructor burnout. Burnout is a response to chronic stress containing: (1) emotional and/or physical exhaustion, (2) lowered job productivity, and (3) over depersonalization. The reasons causing burnout are multidimensional, encompassing physical, mental, and behavioral com-ponents. Typically, a previously pleasurable activity, teaching aerobic dance, becomes a source of undue stress because the environmental demands (exercise fatigue, number of classes, potential participant injury, and so forth) outweigh the response capability of the instructor. Specifically, too many instructors teach too many classes daily and weekly. They are paid little but have immense job responsibility. The overburdened schedule and responsibility cause emotional and physical exhaustion, chronic injury, decreased level of productivity and efficiency, depression, interpersonal difficulties, and eventual burnout.

Interestingly, many instructors fall into the burnout syndrome because of enthusiasm. They want to teach many classes. They want to share with others, as well as earn money. However, the very nature of instructing aerobic dance and the essential economic structure of the fitness industry causes instructor burnout.

To counteract burnout, an instructor may try the following suggestions.

1. Reduce the number of teaching hours to a maximum of two classes per day. (This may be difficult if trying to support yourself through teaching aerobic dance. Remember that more than two hours a day will surely lead to chronic injury.)
2. Keep the number of participants per class manageable. Too large a number is impossible to teach and monitor.
3. Follow acceptable training guidelines for yourself as well as for participants.

Motivation. Motivation is probably the most important behavioral component for the participant. Unfortunately, many individuals who begin exercise programs drop out because they lack the self-motivation to continue. Obviously, other reasons exist for noncompliance, such as medical problems or lack of support from a spouse. But most reasons for dropping out: too little time to exercise, too busy, too many family demands, and so forth, are indirect results of little self-motivation.

We believe that lack of self-motivation is linked to how much the participant values exercise. Values are those experiences or things in our lives that have worth or satisfy our needs or desires. To value exercise is to believe in its utility and importance. That is, if we believe that exercise fulfills not only our fitness needs but also fulfills our need for fun, individualism, worth, and completeness, we will cherish the act of exercising. Only then will a participant make a lifelong commitment.

Unfortunately, too much worth has been placed on the fitness components of exercise and the resultant change in body composition. A perfect body is not possible if the participant does not have the perfect genetic building blocks to begin with. Exercise can and will make the body toned, lean, and muscular. Perhaps an understanding of basic anatomical structure and genetic make-up can enlighten us about the possibility of having a perfect body.

As we have learned, muscle type, either red or white muscle fibers, are inherited. Exercise cannot change the fiber type. This basic principle applies to muscle and bone structure as well as fat pad depot sites. We inherit our bone and muscle length. We may have long muscles and bones or short muscles and bones. We may have long arms and short legs or short arms and long legs. No amount of exercise will change muscle and bone length. We also inherit the predisposition of depot site from our parents. Some of us have a predisposition to lay down fat around the abdomen. Others have a predisposition to lay down fat pads in our thighs and hips. Still others have more fat pads in the upper chest and bust. That is, some of us are pear shaped, others are round, others angular. These different combinations of body size have been analyzed to form three distinct body types: ectomorph (long muscles and bones, tall, angular, thin shape), mesomorph (medium muscles and bones, medium height, with athletic, muscular shape), and endomorph (short muscles and bones, stocky, fleshy shape). Few if any people could be called a perfect endomorph or ectomorph. Most of us are a little of each, such as an angular upper torso with a stocky lower torso. No amount of exercise can change the genetic disposition of body type. Of course, through exercise, we can make that body type fit and healthy. But, if we do not have the genetic building blocks to be Loni Anderson or Tom Selleck, we will never make the ideal. We have genetic limitations.

We believe participants should understand their limitations but should also celebrate and appreciate their uniqueness. We may not have "gorgeous" bodies, but we can enjoy exercise and make a lifetime commitment to health-related fitness.

Philosophically, we, as people, are not a dichotomy of mind and body. We are not solely body or solely mind. Rather, we are a unity of mind and body. We function as a whole. In exercise, participants should be encouraged to exercise for the value of movement and the pleasure it brings. Participants should not be encouraged to exercise solely for an extrinsic bodily reason: a fit, healthy body. Of course, we should all value good health and fitness because they make our lives effective and efficient. But too much concern for the body denies the mind and spirit. We believe that for fitness to become a lifelong commitment, the participant must value exercise for both its bodily utility and inherent worth.

In order to instill such a value system, the participant must come to appreciate exercise for the enjoyment it brings. As instructors, we can help the participant by making the exercise setting bright and cheery, and the exercise experience fun. Training is difficult, but it need not be tedious. We believe the instructor should focus on the positive side of the exercise and not the negative side of work and pain. If the student realizes the rewards, physically, mentally, and spiritually, of exercise and fitness, they will modify their value system. Exercise will then become an important intrinsic value throughout their lives.

A Final Note.   Good teaching is measured by learning. The more the student learns, the better the teacher. No one style is best; good teaching comes in various styles, but good teachers are invariably organized, enthusiastic, and competent.

Cueing may help participants learn aerobic dance routines, but cueing can be hazardous to the instructor's voice, and may hinder the learning process.

The instructor should be aware that too much involvement in aerobic dance may cause burnout. The instructor would be wise to limit class instruction to twice daily. Motivation for the instructor and participant lies in valuing exercise for both its intrinsic and extrinsic merits. Lifetime commitment is based on a philosophy of health-related fitness for the total being.

chapter

7

Application of Knowledge

AEROBIC DANCE INJURIES AND PREVENTION

Introduction

Research indicates that aerobic dance is spawning an epidemic of exercise injuries, especially among instructors. Injury rates for participants are as high as 43 percent and as low as 30 percent, and for instructors as high as 76 percent and as low as 30 percent. Because of the manner in which most programs operate, it's not surprising that instructors have a high injury rate. In a vast majority of commercial fitness programs, a number of very fit young women are the aerobic dance instructors. They work for low wages and teach numerous classes, sometimes four a day, four to six days a week. Because of the ballistic, percussive nature of impact aerobics, they are suffering accumulated stresses that equal running 60 to 100 miles a week. These stresses are resulting in a variety of stress-related injuries. These stresses can be lowered through management of floor construction and surface, shoe selection, and choreography content and style (low-impact aerobics). But, too many injuries are the direct result of doing too much.

However, overuse may not be the sole cause of aerobic dance injury since participants are also suffering injury even though they are participating at safe levels—the standard is 45 minutes a session, three to four sessions a week, which includes 20 minutes of warm-up and cool-down per session. Apparently, other factors beside overuse are causing participant injury, such as muscular imbalance and instant trauma.

But before we continue further, we need a basic understanding of injury categories in sports-related activity. These categories are: instant trauma, mechanical problems, and overuse syndrome.

Categories of Injuries

Instant Trauma.   Instant trauma is any injury that immediately or instantly occurs, such as a sprain, a strain, or a sudden blow. A sprain is a tearing or stretching of ligamentous tissue usually occurring when a joint is twisted beyond its normal range of motion. Ligaments are the stabilizers of joints; if you sprain a ligament, joint instability may occur. For example, the most common sprain is rolling the ankle laterally or outward. The result is tenderness, swelling, and discoloration along the lateral malleolus (ankle bone). Immediate care is RICE. RICE, the first letter of REST, ICE, COMPRESSION and ELEVATION, should be followed to expedite injury recuperation.

Rest is immobilization of the injured site to decrease irritation and edema (fluid retention). Any injury needs time to heal itself. Ice represents ice massage of the injury at intervals of not more than 10 minutes per session or ice bag application for not more than 30 minutes. Ice massage or ice bag application reduces pain and modifies the acute inflammation by (1) vasoconstriction (constricting the blood vessels), (2) reducing muscle temperature, and (3) acting as an analgesic. Ice massage should continue up to 72 hours after injury and be applied before and after use, if exercise must occur.

Compression is restriction of the injury through use of elastic bandages. Compression reduces fluid retention at the site. Edema occurs at an injury to immobilize or splint the injury. Unfortunately, edema causes loss of flexibility and pain when tissue is distended through increased fluid retention. Through compression, edema is modified and pain is lessened. Generally, compression should continue as long as swelling or tenderness is present.

Elevation is raising the injured site above the heart to restrict blood flow and decrease fluid retention. Elevation is simply resting the injury by taking weight off and raising it. Anyone can practice elevation wherever they may be. Specifically, RICE helps reduce the acute inflammatory phase which is the classic swelling, redness, burning, and pain.

Recuperation for a sprain can be anywhere from a week to twelve weeks, depending on the severity of injury. A total rupture of ligamentous tissue usually requires surgical intervention. If extreme tenderness or pain persists, see a physician.

A strain is a tearing or stretching of muscle or tendon fibers that can be a result of an instant trauma or a mechanical imbalance. For example, lifting too great a load or putting too much force on a muscle can result in a strain. A strain results in tenderness, swelling, functional inability to use the muscle, and possible discoloration. Recuperation is typically one to six weeks. Immediate care for a strain is RICE. If extreme pain, swelling, and inability to use the muscle persists, see a physician.

Mechanical Problems. The second category of injury is mechanical problems such as muscular inflexibility or imbalance. Muscular imbalances or inflexibility can cause moderate to severe tendon or muscle tears. Because muscles have an adequate blood supply, any internal muscle injury will usually heal itself in approximately six weeks. In contrast, tendons have little blood supply, and healing is a slow process. Typically, mechanical problems cause nagging muscle and tendon soreness such as persistent low back pain. These mechanical problems can be alleviated by correcting the inefficiency. In contrast, if a tendon is torn from its insertion, the tendon must be surgically reattached and recuperation is typically one year from the time of the injury. Immediate care for mechanical problems is RICE. Beyond that, the mechanical imbalance must be remedied. Mechanical problems should only be diagnosed by physicians, physical therapists, or other qualified health professionals. Some current aerobic dance specialists are promoting guidelines to monitor and diagnose mechanical imbalance problems in participants. We believe that such diagnostic skills must be left to certified, trained medical personnel. If the instructor suspects that a chronic injury or pain is due to poor mechanical alignment, the instructor should refer the participant to qualified health professionals.

Overuse Syndrome. Overuse injury typically occurs in bone or soft tissue. This injury is suffered by athletes, dancers, and now aerobic exercisers who, through repetitive activity, place too much stress on tissue and bone. Too much stress on a bone may result in a stress fracture, which is an actual small fracture of the bone. Stress fractures often occur in the lower leg as the direct result of the ballistic and percussive forces of the body as it jumps, hops, runs, gallops, and skips. The body takes off, flies, and then lands. As the foot meets the floor, force is absorbed through the shoe, foot, ankle, lower leg, knee, and so on. Through repetitive forces, the bone tries to remodel itself along the lines of increased stress. The constant repetitive stresses lead to muscle fatigue. As fatigue develops, a loss of shock absorption occurs. The pain increases and disuse of the area causes further muscle atrophy or decrease in size. The cycle continues, and if rest does not occur, a stress fracture results. If the force is not absorbed correctly or too much force is repetitively applied, the bone is weakened at one specific site and a pinpoint fracture occurs. Recuperation for stress fractures is usually four to eight weeks.

Soft tissue injury occurs to connective tissue such as tendons, the bursa (a fluid-filled sac surrounding a joint that enables tendons to slide smoothly across the joint), or nonmuscular tissue such as fascia, the connective tissue surounding a muscle. The injury happens in much the same manner as a stress fracture. Repetitive forces cause an irritation to the connective tissue which predisposes an inflammation. The result is tendonitis, bursitis, or even fasciitis. Unfortunately, soft tissue injuries heal at a very slow rate, almost twice as slow as a stress fracture. Typically a soft tissue injury may require up to twelve weeks for recovery. Recovery time is dependent on: age and immediate management of the injury.

The immediate management for stress fractures and soft tissue injury is, once again, RICE. In addition, the training program must be changed and mechanical abnormalities corrected. Unfortunately, most athletes as well as aerobic dance instructors are their own worst enemies in training and injury recovery. The injured instructor will deny that she is injured and refuse to rest. We have seen too many instructors with soft tissue injury who continue to exercise even though in pain. Typically, instructors argue that they are resting since the injured limb is used only during aerobics class. They also say, "I have to teach my class, and as soon as class is over, I will not do anything until my next class." However, the continued use in class and daily normal use will have an exponential effect on the injury. The more use, the greater the time until the site is healed.

Reducing Injury Potential

The potential for instant trauma can be lowered by following a safe and sound exercise protocol. For example, do not exercise when tired. Fatigue slows reaction time and increases the potential for instant trauma. Also, clear the floor surface of loose debris, projecting floor boards, or any other outcropping that might catch your foot. The floor surface should not encumber movement. A sticky, soft, or carpeted floor will have a higher injury potential through catching the foot and turning the ankle. Insure that participants and instructors have plenty of room to move, and that no wall outcroppings exist. Each aerobic dance participant should have a minimum of 8 to 10 square feet of floor space. An exercise room that violates space requirements for each participant will increase instant trauma potential with individuals inevitably striking each other. The choice of shoes will also decrease ankle injury potential. The shoe should be suitably constructed with support stitching across the metatarsals. If participants have a history of ankle sprains, they should first strengthen the muscles surrounding the ankle to increase stability. Second, they should wear a shoe that has plenty of support.

Injuries from inadequate flexibility and muscle imbalance can be decreased through a complete, health-related fitness program. The majority of low back pain is related to poor rectus abdominus muscle strength and inadequate low back and hamstring muscle flexibility. Flexibility can be increased through slow, overload stretching of each joint. Flexibility was discussed in Chapter 2, along with examples of flexibility exercises.

Muscle imbalance can be improved through a complete strength training program for all seven major muscle groups. See Chapter 2 for information concerning strength training. Many muscle tears occur because one muscle is too strong in relation to its antagonistic (the opposite) muscle.

For example, a football wide receiver sprints to catch a thrown pass. His quadricep muscles are too strong in relation to the hamstring muscles and the hamstrings are stretched beyond their normal range of motion. The muscle tears and an injury occurs. This injury can be avoided by developing the quadriceps at a 3 to 2 ratio to the hamstrings. Most other muscles and their reciprocals can be developed at a 1 to 1 ratio, which means developing muscular strength and endurance in each muscle group equally.

Overuse injuries are the direct result of (1) overuse, (2) inadequate floor construction, (3) poor quality shoes, (4) inadequate and incompetent instruction, (5) inherited structural weakness or muscular imbalance, and (6) age.

(1) Overuse in High-Impact Aerobics.   Because of the repetitive nature of dance routines, high-impact aerobics can be the culprit for overuse syndrome. Usually, aerobic dances are choreographed with a majority of stepping occurring on the ball of the foot whether jumping, hopping, running, skipping, or galloping. Because the body is actually flying through space, the force must be absorbed by the lower body when it lands. These forces radiate through the lower leg and stress the tibia, fibula, and all other connective soft tissue. Because most aerobic dance instructors and some participants exercise too much, the body is unable to control the inflammation process. Inflammation occurs with accompanying discomfort.

In our studies we have found that a common aerobic dance step such as a step, hop, step, kick performed for 15 seconds has almost 5 times the accumulated force compared to an athlete jumping for height as many times as possible in 15 seconds. Others have found that aerobic dancers performing the pony suffer accumulated stress three times the body weight in vertical, multiple, and unilateral force. Obviously, there are many variables that affect these results. But specifically, we believe that the lateral and unilateral forces associated with the repetitiveness of impact aerobic dance initiate high levels of accumulated stress.

In order to counteract overuse, we recommend a few commonsense rules:

A. Do not engage in high-impact aerobics more than 20 minutes a session, three times a week.
B. If you need more aerobic exercise a week, participate in a low-impact weight bearing activity such as low-impact aerobics or walking.
C. If suffering from a stress injury, find an alternative nonweight bearing activity, such as swimming, bicycling, or rowing machines, that give the cell-repairing process an opportunity to reduce the inflammation. Do not continue to stress the injury with any activity that places additional weight against the injury site. Do not continue in a weightlifting program that irritates the injured site, because lifting gives additional stress and load.
D. If you have a history of soft tissue injury, or joint inflammation, do not enter a high-impact aerobics class. We wonder if low-impact aerobics are acceptable since weight bearing is occurring on the injured limb. Also, remember that running is a high-impact activity even though the accumulated stresses are less than aerobic dance. Running or any ballistic, percussive, high-impact activity will create the same type of stress as excessive aerobic dance. We would recommend that you participate in swimming, walking, biking or rowing, but remember that too much of a good thing can cause similar soft tissue injury. Moderation above all things. If you want or need to do more aerobic activities, we recommend a varied program of low-impact activity interspersed with nonimpact activities.

(2) Inadequate Floor Construction.   Injury is also related to the type of floor surface. Many descriptive studies have reported that concrete covered with a pad or carpet has the highest injury rate. The second highest injury rate occurs with wood over airspace, or wood over airspace with a padded cover. Because high-impact aerobics places great stress on the body, especially the lower leg, floors should be constructed to help absorb the forces.

Unfortunately, very few facilities have a floor that reduces joint stress. Most facilities have carpet laid over a subflooring such as concrete, or maybe carpet on plywood on concrete, which is the equivalent of running on asphalt. We know that runners have always suffered from stress injuries, and many running tracks are now designed to be more resilient, but aerobic dancing puts a greater stress on soft tissue. As a runner lands, the stresses are distributed across the foot from the heel to the ball. This is different from high-impact aerobics, where the force is limited to the ball of the foot.

To decrease stress levels and injury, the aerobic dance flooring should have resiliency. The flooring situation is not a complicated issue. Two basic types of flooring, either a padded floor or a spring/suspension floor, should be used for aerobic dance.

A suspension floor is constructed of an absorbent, resilient pad laid to cover the total area between the base floor and a finished floor covering. A spring floor is constructed of coiled springs, installed proportionately apart between the base floor and a subfloor, topped by a finished floor. A padded system covers either a hardwood surface or concrete, usually about three-quarters of an inch thick. The padding is of good absorbent and resilient quality and covered with a finished product.

The major stumbling block for many fitness centers is the expense of a suspended/spring or padded floor. However, the expense is justified considering the injury potential of a nonresilient surface. A padded floor with a finished surface is less expensive but may not wear as well as the spring or suspension floor. And, padded floors probably should be limited to aerobic or exercise classes. Due to the absorbency of the pad, be aware that absorbency and resilience are not the only factors to consider when using a padded floor. Twisting and turning motions should be limited on a padded surface due to the torque or movement of forces that cause rotation. The pronation of the foot and leg, and the degree of torque can potentially cause severe injuries. Any such movement should be avoided on a padded surface. When a padded mat system is purchased, find out how absorbent the surface is. How does it respond to the shock of the body hitting the surface? How often will it be used? How impervious is it to moisture, such as body perspiration? If the floor is not moisture resistant, an accumulation of body sweat and skin sloughs will create smell and decay. How long before the product begins to break down and bend at the edges?

Spring floors have a greater adaptability because they are useful in gymnastics or other rebound activities. And, a suspension floor is ideal for basketball or volleyball. The type of floor you select should address: (a) the absorbency and resiliency factor, (b) its durability, and (c) its ability to meet other activity needs.

(3) Poor Quality Shoes.   The type of shoe worn in aerobic dance can also affect injury occurrence. Because of the biomechanical difference between running and hopping/jumping, which is the prevalent motion in aerobic dance, a running shoe will not serve the purpose. Running shoes are designed to handle a heel-strike impact, not the lateral stresses or the abundance of vertical stresses that are involved in most aerobic dance programs. Research studies show that shoes do absorb up to 10 percent of forces suffered by the body, hence, a good quality shoe is necessary. Obviously, a shoe is imperative even though we have seen people participate without them. No one should ever participate in an impact activity without durable, quality shoes.

Because of the unique lateral and vertical stresses of aerobic dance, the aerobic shoe should have extra stitching across the metatarsals to prevent the foot from rolling (Figure 7-1, p. 152). Extra padding at the sole should cover the ball of the foot to help defer the vertical stresses. The heel should be reinforced to give extra support. However, most aerobic dancers want a shoe that is lightweight, which is a difficult request. For a shoe to give the absorbency needed, it must have more weight.

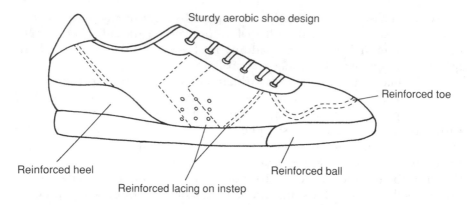

Good shoes are expensive, and unfortunately aerobic shoes have a short durability life. Depending on the amount of use, an aerobic shoe can become worthless in two to three months. If the shoe has lost its form and the soles are becoming worn, discard them.

Anatomical abnormalities, foot pronation, and so forth are continual sources for mechanical problems. We recommend a visit to a sports podiatrist first to find the best shoe. For one visit the cost may be as much as $60 to $90. However, if injury occurs because of an imbalance, the cost for a physical therapist may be $40 per visit. If exercise is going to occur, make an investment in quality shoes.

(4) Inadequate or Incompetent Instruction.   The rapid increase of aerobic dance has meant that anybody with a tape deck and a few borrowed steps can be an instructor. Typically, instructors are young, fit, beautiful, and look great in skimpy leotards. Even if the instructor is an experienced dancer, this is no guarantee of competency.

Most employers do not expect much of their instructors beyond being trim, fit, beautiful, energetic, and enthusiastic. Instructors are not expected to know anatomy, physiology, or exercise technique. The result is young, fit, beautiful women leading unfit, middle-aged, overweight women in exercises that probably neither should be doing. Many injuries occur because of poor exercise technique and just plain ignorance on the instructor's part. We cannot fault the instructors, because they disseminate their limited education. The employers are partially at fault since they refuse to pay a decent wage to hire competent instructors. Instructors are viewed as "throwaways" who are hired at low wages, worked excessive hours, and then laid off when injured. At the same time, employers get away with this practice because participants do not demand quality instruction. Instead, most participants want the cheapest exercise program possible. Cheap programs promulgate cheap instruction. An employer cannot afford to hire an educated exercise specialist so they hire the young, fit, incompetent instructor. Unfortunately, for the consumer/participant it is becoming more difficult to find out if the instructor is incompetent. Most instructors are now certified through some agency, but certifications are typically given after only two days of intensive study. As exercise professionals with many years study, we find such certification processes an insult to exercise science. Certification should be a continuing process and instructors should spend time in competent inservice programs. Unless an instructor has knowledge concerning exercise, they should not be teaching others about exercise. (For more on certification, see Chapter 9.)

Inadequate instruction can result in instant trauma as well as overuse syndrome. Instant trauma and injuries caused by mechanical problems can be eliminated by following acceptable exercise guidelines and developing adequate strength and flexibility levels (see Chapters 2, 3, 4, and 5). Overuse syndrome can be decreased by keeping the frequency of impact aerobics to not more than three times a week, with each session limited to 20 minutes of actual aerobics. Overuse can also be decreased by modifying the dance steps. We often see instructors who admonish their participants to kick higher, jump higher, and so on. Unfortunately, that kicking higher multiplies the joint stress. It is true that more cardiovascular work occurs with a higher kick but the cardiovascular intensity is not worth the extra joint stress. Choreography should be limited to low to moderate leg kicking, jumping, or hopping.

Low-impact aerobics, always keeping one foot on the floor, can decrease stress markedly by almost 900 percent (stress platforms, mechanical plates that measure forces, have verified the magnified stresses of high-impact aerobic dance), because the body is not flying and less joint stress is absorbed by the lower leg. Typically, low-impact aerobics incorporates more arm exercise in order to raise the heart to working effect. Routines are composed of sliding, walking, knee raises, and so forth, done with counterbalance arm motion. The heart rate is raised to the working range through a coordinated, whole-body workout. However, low-impact aerobics can also cause joint stress if movements are not kept in control. Frantic arm swings and overuse of the ligamentous, tendon tissue in the shoulder, elbow, and wrist can also cause soft tissue injury. The best advice is to keep all motion under control and limit the repetitiveness of motion to three times a week. (See Chapter 5 for discussion of choreography techniques.)

We have also seen many instructors use hand or ankle weights to improve their workout. We doubt and question the acceptability of using hand weights in an aerobic dance program except in isolated muscle strengthening programs. Cardiovascular intensity is increased with hand or ankle weights, but the joint stress multiplies. If you want a greater load for your workout, give yourself some more time. Remember, intensity, duration, and frequency are the elements for a good workout. (If you need a review, reread Chapters 1 and 2.)

(5) Inherited Structural Weakness or Muscular Imbalance. We have already discussed inherited structural and muscular imbalance. Specifically, remember that an aerobic dance instructor is not competent to diagnose such problems. If any of your clients are suffering continual strains or sprains or complain of low back pain or foot pain, refer them to competent medical personnel.

(6) Age. None of us enjoy growing older and having to accept physical limitations. Nothing is going to stop the aging process. We can slow and buffer aging through good exercise, rest, nutrition, weight control, and stress reduction, but we cannot stop the process. This does not mean that we cannot improve as we grow older. Regular vigorous physical activity does produce physiological improvement regardless of age. But, the magnitude of the changes depends on several factors, including initial fitness status, age, and the specific type of training. It appears that older individuals are not able to improve their strength and endurance capacity to the same extent as younger people. This is probably because of a general decline in neuromuscular function, as well as an age-related impairment in the cell's capability for protein synthesis and chemical regulation.

This means that as we age, all physiological processes slow, including the healing process. Also, we become more susceptible to injury from overuse syndrome, muscular imbalance, and instant trauma. By following a sensible, acceptable exercise program, we should not suffer undue injury. However, perhaps we need to understand that some forms of exercise should be limited, especially impact aerobic activities. This does not mean that we should stop exercising. On the contrary, we should continue vigorous, aerobic exercise, but perhaps the exercise mode should be swimming, bicycling, cross country skiing, walking, and so forth.

We personally believe that middle-aged and older women should not participate in impact aerobic dance. We have seen too many injuries that could easily have been avoided through a modified aerobic program. If a participant has no history of stress injuries, has no problem with accidental urination, and can jump rope for two minutes a day for seven days, then she or he probably can begin an aerobic dance program. However, perhaps swimming or walking would be a better choice. If participants have a long history of aerobic dance exercise with no problems, they probably can continue, though we would recommend an alternative program to high-impact aerobics.

How to Avoid Aerobic Dance Injuries

To avoid and prevent aerobic dance injury, we recommend that you (1) Limit impact aerobic exercise to three times a week, at twenty minutes per aerobic session, (2) Only aerobic dance on an absorbent or resilient floor, (3) Wear only quality foot wear; replace shoes when worn, and see a sport podiatrist, (4) If you are the aerobic dance instructor, increase your knowledge through continued inservice classes, (5) Be leery of enrolling middle-aged women in your aerobic dance classes if they have never aerobically exercised before. (Have these people jump rope, one minute a day for one week. If they have no discomfort after one week, they can probably aerobic dance with no adverse affects), (6) If you incur a soft tissue injury, or a joint becomes tender, follow prescribed injury management techniques, (7) Ensure that all participants have enough room to move, 10 feet square minimum, (8) Ensure that no outcroppings from the walls in your facility exist, and (9) Keep your floor surfaces clean and free from any debris.

What to Do If an Injury Occurs

We recommend that anyone teaching a physical activity class be certified in CPR and advanced first aid. In fact, any reputable agency will not certify aerobic dance instructors without CPR certification. Any potential life-threatening situation could occur in an exercise class. In our years of exercise training and teaching, we have seen many freak injuries occur that technically should not have happened. To offer first aid, the aerobic instructor must know what is acceptable treatment. Generally, for the typical sprains and strains that occur in aerobic dance, RICE is the best immediate care. The best care is over care; have a physician evaluate and diagnose the injury. Aerobic dance instructors are not qualified to decide the severity of an injury.

Is the Instructor Liable?

Unfortunately, that answer is "yes". My statements reflect what exercise professionals should always follow in establishing any program. For an attorney's perspective of liability, see Chapter 8.

First, hiring a sports medicine professional is important to assist your staff in developing routines for your aerobics classes. Document in writing how the sports medicine professional contributed to and approved the program.

Second, have the program evaluated periodically by a professional consultant in sports medicine. If sued, present the court with documented evidence of how the program has taken the utmost care and responsibility in developing exercise programs, choreography, and so forth.

Hire only well-rounded, qualified instructors. Even if the instructors are experienced and qualified, an instructor training program should be developed for your facility. Preferably, this training program should be verified and put in writing by a sports medicine professional. Develop a manual that follows general guidelines regarding injury protection and requires instructors to be certified through an acceptable agency. To remain current, instructors should demonstrate professionalism through attendance at inservice workshops and professional organizations.

If you choose to avoid hiring a sports medicine professional to approve your program development, do not show your ignorance. If any unsound advice is printed, you and your facility's liability will increase.

Education is an important aspect in any exercise facility. Periodically give class participants printed or typed handouts containing information concerning injury prevention, exercise prescription, and so forth. But again, ensure that the information is correct, and avoid exercises that are considered controversial by sports medicine professionals.

Every exercise professional should seriously consider requiring each participant, whether a member or just a guest, to read and sign a written disclaimer and release form. The form should disclaim any liability for negligence on the part of you and your facility. The release should also describe the nature of the aerobic dance program, and request that each person consult a physician prior to participation.

At the very least, the release should require that the participant acknowledge the potential for aerobic injury; a statement by the participant that he or she agrees to be solely responsible for any injuries sustained as a result of his or her participation; and a statement that the participant agrees to hold blameless the facility, the staff, and instructor for any injuries incurred while using the facility.

Consult an attorney to prepare your release to ensure that the language is prepared according to your state or local laws. Probably the best protection against lawsuit liability is to buy liability insurance. The insurance cost is small in relation to the peace of mind it gives you.

How to Avoid Being Sued

To avoid being sued, it becomes imperative to follow acceptable exercise guidelines developed by reputable sports medicine organizations, such as the American College of Sports Medicine. Generally their position recommends quantity and quality of training for developing and maintaining cardiovascular fitness and body composition in adults.

Second, become certified through a quality certification program. Ensure that the certifying agency has developed specific standards. Specifically, they should require a written test to evaluate exercise science knowledge, a fitness test to measure personal fitness, a practical test to evaluate choreography and exercise standards knowledge, and a demand for CPR certification. Also, the aerobic dance certification should have an expiration date that forces updating and renewal.

Third, keep updated in your training whenever the opportunity arises, and implement that knowledge in your exercise routines. Keep receipts and document your certification and participation in such programs.

Fourth, be sure you follow prescribed warm-up protocols accepted by sports medicine professionals (see Chapters 1 and 2). The slow, rhythmic warm-up movement should increase blood flow throughout the body. This should be followed by a head to foot slow, static stretching program.

Fifth, explain what you are doing when you are leading exercise and aerobic dance routines. Explain what is proper technique, what is improper technique, and why. If someone is performing something wrong, teach them the correct method and explain why. Be a professional at all times. Educate your participants and help them understand the importance of their being responsible for their own exercise actions. If an exercise is difficult or causes discomfort, they should investigate why. They should be educated to become discriminating consumers concerning their exercise programs. No one should blindly follow exercise personnel who are teaching incorrect or potentially dangerous exercise techniques.

A Final Note

Activity injuries, as well as aerobic dance injuries, can be prevented by following acceptable training procedures. If an injury occurs, RICE (Rest, Ice, Constriction, Elevation) is the immediate management technique to follow. For aerobic dance instructors, education, certification, and acceptable training techniques are the guidelines for avoiding participant injury and limiting liability.

.

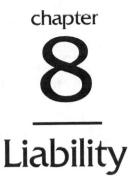

chapter

8

Liability

Mark S. Moorer, J.D.

INTRODUCTION

The author's goal throughout this text has been to educate the reader. My goal in this chapter is to inform the reader of some basic problems confronting fitness entrepreneurs who either teach, train, or own a fitness business, and any combination thereof. Specifically, problems whose ultimate remedy is the legal system. I will not delve deeply into the topic areas. Instead, my purpose is to acquaint the reader with enough information to enable you to recognize legal liability.

The subsequent material is not intended to and does not constitute legal advice. If legal questions arise, find counsel and seek advice. Every jurisdiction is unique and the material offered in this text is generic. Readers who have specific questions or problems should consult an attorney if any resolution is to be found.

Do not underestimate the scope of your legal liability. No one is immune from legal liability. Legal questions can arise immediately as you first venture into the fitness business, beginning with resolving what activities will be offered and what kind of business form will be established.

Type and Number of Fitness Business

There are three generally accepted business forms: sole proprietorship, partnerships, and corporate formations.

Sole Proprietorship.   A sole proprietorship is a business owned and operated for the pleasure of one person. It is in every respect the alter ego of that individual. Therefore, that individual is totally responsible for the acts committed by that business, and on behalf of that business by its employees.

Partnership.   In contrast, a partnership is an association of two or more persons as co-owners for a profit. This business form is presumably more solvent than a proprietorship because more accumulated assets cover the potential business liability. However, just like a proprietorship, the partners are ultimately, jointly responsible for the actions of the business.

Corporations.   As an alternative, many individuals like to shield themselves from liability by forming a corporation. A corporation is a legal entity, created in accordance with legal statutes in a particular state. A corporation is separate and distinct from the persons who own its stock. Therefore, when a corporation is formed, the people forming the corporation may work within the corporation with limited liability. The separateness of entities is the key.

Limiting Liability by Business Form.   The purpose of this discussion should be clear. One method of reducing exposure to legal action is by forming a business structure which reduces business risk. Thus, even if sued, and even if the plaintiff prevails, personal exposure is reduced if one is operating within the corporate form. Why? Because the corporate assets are distinct and separate from personal assets. In the sole proprietorship and partnership form, one's exposure includes personal assets to cover losses. See an attorney, who will help explain these possibilities and the extrinsic costs in initiating a formation decision.

No matter what business form is developed, the form will have a nominal effect on legal liability. A business owner needs to worry about adequacy of facilities and competency of instructors more than anything else. Most lawsuits arise from these two issues.

Safe and Adequate Facilities

When an exercise business invites participants onto the business property, the owners are charged with the legal duty to use reasonable and ordinary care in keeping the property reasonably safe. The general duty includes

1. warning the participants of any concealed or dangerous conditions that the owner knows exist,
2. providing ordinary care in active operation on the property, plus
3. having a duty to make reasonable inspections to discover any dangerous conditions, and thereafter
4. making those dangerous conditions safe.

Perhaps an illustration may be helpful. Imagine a fitness facility where cushioned mats are used for aerobic exercise. The mats are used to cushion impact. However, only a portion of the floor is covered, the general area where the participants exercise. A participant drifts out of the general area, trips over a raised mat edge, and twists an ankle. Is the owner liable? Maybe.

The landowner owes participants the duty to inform them of the dangerous mat condition and probably is required to make the mat condition safe, that is, matting the whole floor. Obviously, this is a simplified example and an attorney would need to prove much more to extend liability to the landowner. However, our point is that a complete assessment must be made to discover any possible dangers within the exercise facility.

Assess the facilities, then inform an attorney about the perceived dangers. Determine if corrections are needed to make the conditions safe. Possibly, the money spent on preventive measures will be well spent in contrast to a lawsuit.

Remember that this is only one way a landowner can incur liability. Another inherent risk is having ultrahazardous equipment, like a mini-tramp. This equipment is ultrahazardous because of the frequency of injury associated with its use — no matter how much care is exercised. If you are intending to use such equipment, or are using the equipment presently, be sure all steps have been taken to make its use as safe as possible. Then, evaluate whether the risk is necessary given the availability of other fitness alternatives.

Finally, remember the authors' point about adequately designed facilities. Profit-maximization is the goal of most if not all businessmen. Sometimes shortcuts are taken to increase facility use by overcrowding or overusing for profits' sake.

However, structures are designed with a fixed limit for participant use at any given time. Any usage above this level increases the risk of injury and proportionately the risk of liability. Don't cheat on the safety of others. It's bad for business and will ultimately cause a legal web that only the courts will unravel.

Fitness Managers

The same concept extends to the person or persons who operate and manage the fitness facility. Hire qualified individuals for the position. Legal exposure arises faster on this issue than any other. Liability can occur from numerous avenues.

What Is Liability?   Liability in human activity refers to being held responsible for negligence.

What Is Negligence?   Negligence is usually the failure to act in some prescribed manner under certain circumstances. To extend liability, a plaintiff must show the existence of a duty on the part of the defendant to conform to a specific standard of conduct for the protection of the plaintiff against an unreasonable risk or injury. The duty owed to the defendant must be breached. The breach of duty must result in the actual and proximate cause of a plaintiff's injury or damage to the plaintiff's person or property.

A general duty of care is imposed on all human activity. When engaged in any human activity, we are under a legal duty to act as an ordinary, prudent, reasonable person. It is presumed that an ordinary person will take reasonable precautions against creating risk. Thus, if a defendant's conduct creates an unreasonable risk of injury to persons in the position of the plaintiff, the general duty of care extends from the defendant to the plaintiff.

For example, the owner of a fitness facility has a duty to hire competent instructors. If an unqualified instructor's teaching leads to and results in an injury to a participant, the owner may well have created an unreasonable risk. The reasonable act of hiring qualified instructors would have avoided this risk. Therefore, the owner breached his/her duty of care. Again, many more variables are involved, but the general implication should be apparent. Hiring unqualified instructors is risky business.

Even if a qualified instructor is hired, liability is not eliminated. Liability may be extended by such factors as the status of the parties or a specific statutory provision of a particular state. Some persons are held to a standard of conduct different from that of the ordinary person.

A person who is a professional with special skill, e.g., a physician, is required to possess and exercise the knowledge and skill of a member of the profession in good standing in the same or similar localities. The professional must also use such superior judgment, skill, and knowledge as he or she actually possesses. Thus if a certified aerobic instructor (presumably a specialist) is hired, who does not exercise that superior skill, the employer may be held liable for the instructor's wrong via the theory of neligent supervision of that employee. The plaintiff has not only the instructor to sue but also the instructor's employer, who will probably be held accountable under the theory of joint and vicarious liability. Simply put, the plaintiff can collect one sum from one, either, or both.

Planning and Liability

The importance of thoughtfully planning the type of fitness enterprise should be apparent. Not only does planning affect the pure cost of developing a facility to house the fitness activities, but planning also affects equipment and activities offered the public, as well as the training and skill level of the supervisors and instructors. A delicate balance must be struck which requires a thorough analysis of all potential problems.

For example, let's assume that money is no object in opening a fitness facility. A modern, super-automated fitness facility is built with highly trained supervisors and instructors. The doors are opened for business. Advertisements state that anyone who enrolls and follows the proscribed fitness program will be in perfect shape within one year.

Inadvertently, the advertisement may have provided a participant with a consumer protection claim, that is, false advertising. Let's say a participant, Joe Smith, no matter how hard he tried, never did get into perfect shape, maybe because his anatomical construction and metabolism would not lend itself to perfection. The advertisements created an expectation of perfection in Joe's mind which presumably was reasonable, but Joe could not achieve it. He wants damages for the money he expended, as well as the emotional trauma resulting from not being able to achieve the perfect body.

This illustration is useful to reinforce the importance of preventive planning, but it also reveals how many avenues must be covered to diminish the probability of legal liability.

Other Issues

Previously in this text, the authors talked about the importance of developing a good screening procedure. I heartily concur. Knowing the participants thoroughly will help prevent injury and limit liability.

The authors also referred to the use of consent forms and liability waivers. Consent forms are obviously good tools for explaining program goals and informing participants of the potential dangers. However, realize that the form only performs that function and in no way limits the duties owed to the participant. The instructor, supervisor, and owner must still act as reasonable, prudent persons would act under similar circumstances.

Further, the liability waiver may explicitly state that the participant will hold harmless the owner if an injury results, but don't count on it. The forms are narrowly construed by most courts. Courts interpret ambiguities against the drafter. The defendant may have to prove that the participant, the plaintiff, meant to waive his or her rights in the specific instance, and so forth. Any bright lawyer can almost summarily get these waivers tossed out of court, usually because courts abhor a forfeiture of rights. This does not mean the waiver and consent form is no good. Not having a form is foolish. Just realize that they have a very limited effect.

A Final Note on Liability

Remember the importance of planning. Determine the type of market needed and develop the facilities to accommodate the market. Make sure the facility is safe for the participant. Use equipment that the participants and staff can use safely and has a low risk associated with it.

Put together a well-qualified staff. Develop a good screening program as well as good fitness programs. Have instructors follow the programs and make sure they are supervised. If instructors deviate from the prescribed program, the owner is at risk. Have participants execute consent forms as well as liability waivers. If all of these concerns are met, the chances of ending up in court are minimal.

Collateral Legal Issues in Fitness Facilities

Two collateral matters for fitness instructors and owners are: liability insurance and possible copyright violations.

Liability Insurance. Liability insurance is very important, simply because it allows many business people to sleep at night without worrying that their entire life's effort will be financially wiped out by one unfortuitous event.

Speak with an attorney about the kind of policy limits you need.

Copyright Violation. First, copyright law is one of the few accepted areas wherein a lawyer can be and should be a specialist. I do not pretend to be such a specialist. For any particular copyright questions, secure the services of a specialist in copyright law. Second, when something is copyrighted it gives the holder of the copyright the exclusive use of that creation. Normally, when the holder allows a third party to use the material, he or she charges a royalty. If an aerobic dance instructor, supervisor, or owner uses the creation of a copyrighted material (taped or recorded copyrighted music) without the creator's permission, the law has been violated, and the violators are subject to legal liability.

To avoid liability, consult with an attorney about acquiring a public performance license from a performing rights society. Two such societies which represent most composers, lyricists, and publishers in the United States are: the American Society of Composers, Authors and Publishers and the Broadcast Music, Inc.

Narrow exceptions to acquiring a license are available. One is material used in nonprofit education institutions.

A Final Note

Every state has different statutes and laws; secure an attorney to help develop your fitness program. Remember to follow acceptable professional guidelines as to facilities, equipment, and hiring practices; using common sense and acceptable practices will decrease your chances of being sued.

chapter

9

Special Considerations

CERTIFICATION PROGRAMS

This final chapter is concerned with special situations in aerobic dance instruction. The chapter is divided into two sections: Certification and Guidelines for Pregnant Participants in Aerobic Dance.

Certification

For aerobic dance, certification is relatively new, starting within the last eight to ten years. However, we wonder about the worth of many aerobic dance certification programs. Specifically, the purpose of certification is to guarantee that the aerobic dance instructor has met a specific standard. The standard should be one comparable to a specific level of knowledge, both practical and theoretical, that guarantees the instructor is competent and effective. This sounds good; an instructor has met specific criteria set forth by an agency and has been certified as having that specific knowledge. Unfortunately, certifying agencies are not equal in what they present or expect for certification. Most agencies present a 2 to 3 day training session followed by an examination. We doubt that such a protocol can prepare an instructor adequately for teaching in any exercise program. We also believe that such certifications provide instructors with just enough information to be dangerous. It is not possible to prepare an adequate and competent professional in a few short hours.

However, certification programs are better than nothing, as long as the instructor realizes the limitations of such programs. The instructor should also evaluate the merits of the certifying agency and the level of preparation needed to pass certification requirements. As you remember from Chapter 8, certification may hold the instructor to a higher standard of professional care. That is, if the instructor is sued, the criteria to measure performance will be by that higher standard. If certification is important, make sure the program is the best that can be offered and is supported by competent sports medicine personnel.

The instructor should also realize that certification will not make a poor instructor into an excellent teacher. Certification is not the answer to all problems in aerobic dance instruction. Some very fine aerobic dance teachers have never been certified. In comparison, some mediocre teachers have certification. Certification only means the instructor has met the merits of a specific agency. In fact, certification only addresses one of the five elements that we discussed throughout this text:

> Committed to fitness
> Educated as a teacher
> Skilled as a teacher
> Competent and able to apply knowledge and skill
> Certification

The other four elements come with time, determination, training, education, and personality.

Another positive argument for certification is that many fitness businesses require one in order to teach aerobic dance. According to a 1987 *Fitness Management Magazine* reader survey, 39 percent of club managers who responded said they preferred certified instructors and 36 percent require certification.

Another problem with certification is that, although numerous agencies and organizations offer aerobic dance instructor certification, each program is different. At present no universal set of standards exists. That is, each agency presents a different perspective of what an aerobic dance instructor should know or perform. We wonder if such guidelines for standards will ever exist, especially considering the history of competency examinations for exercise and nutrition professionals. Few professional fitness or sport organizations, outside of athletic training, demand certification from qualified programs. For example, just about anyone can become a coach. Employers such as school districts, youth sport programs, and so forth either do not demand or do not know how to evaluate competency. Unfortunately, competency is usually equated with a successful winning program instead of the values taught. The same rule of thumb exists in fitness programs concerning certification for exercise leaders. Obviously, exceptions do exist such as the YMCA and other programs guided by degreed fitness professionals. In contrast, we wonder how many commercial fitness facilities are managed or owned by degreed exercise science personnel. A common set of standards or guidelines will only occur if state legislatures force the issue.

Until that time, if ever, the best advice for an aerobic dance instructor is to learn as much as possible and to become certified. We recommend certification through either the American College of Sport Medicine (ACSM) or the Institute for Aerobic Research. ACSM's aerobic leadership program is a 32-hour course that focuses on teaching skills and physiology. To qualify, the instructor must be certified by some other organization or have 250 hours of teaching experience within the past two years.

Kenneth Cooper's Institute for Aerobic Research offers two 40-hour courses that conclude with a written and practical exam. The Physical Fitness Specialist program focuses on physiology, wellness, and safety, and the Group Exercise Leader program emphasizes classroom skills.

Some other national programs providing certification are International Dance Education Association (IDEA) and Foundation and Aerobics and Fitness Association of America (AFAA). IDEA does not train instructors, but offers a 172-question written exam that tests knowledge of physiology, nutrition, dance program design, and other areas. AFAA offers a 20-hour course in physiology, nutrition, and dance program design, followed by a written and practical exam. AFAA-certified instructors must take continuing education courses to remain current. The organization also presents supplemental courses and certification in specialties like low-impact aerobics and prenatal aerobics.

PREGNANCY AND EXERCISE

Introduction

With the growing awareness of the physiological benefits associated with an aerobic exercise regimen, pregnant women want to exercise—safely. They are interested not only in the usual benefits of aerobic exercise but also the potential for ease of delivery and improved posture.

In the past few years many exercise tapes have been designed for prenatal exercise. Unfortunately, many of these programs are compiled by nonprofessionals with insufficient medical or research information. The American College of Obstetricians and Gynecologists found much information inappropriate, inaccurate, and/or incomplete. Therefore, aerobic instructors working with pregnant women should continually seek further education as to safe exercise routines for these women. Current research is consistently shedding new light on this issue.

Exercise Guidelines

Until recently, established exercise guidelines for pregnant women did not exist. In 1985, the American College of Obstetricians and Gynecologists developed guidelines for exercise during pregnancy (Table 9-1). These guidelines were established for the average pregnant woman and are only recommended training tips and ranges. Each pregnant woman should seek her physician's advice to develop an individualized exercise prescription for her own specific needs. Women who enter pregnancy with a high aerobic fitness capacity may be able to exercise at a greater intensity compared to women with average or low capacities.

Before we can discuss an aerobic conditioning program for pregnant women, we must first examine the basic physiological changes that occur during pregnancy. Norms are unavailable because of the varied individual physiological response to pregnancy. The following changes are only approximations.

Cardiovascular Changes

Cardiac output is the volume of blood pumped by the heart in one minute. The product of heart rate and stroke volume equals cardiac output. Stroke volume is the amount of blood pumped from the left ventricle with one heart beat. Cardiac output increase aproximately 40 percent during the first 10 weeks of pregnancy and remains stable until delivery. The increase occurs because heart rate and stroke volume increase. By the third trimester, a typical heart rate will increase to approximately 85 bpm. Heart rate will increase because of the added weight gain associated with pregnancy. The added weight of pregnancy causes the heart to work harder, therefore possibly increasing stroke volume. Blood volume increases approximately 40 percent because plasma volume expands. Plasma is the liquid portion of the blood. The blood volume probably increases because of the increase in fluid retention. Because red cell volume increases at a slower rate compared to blood volume, hemodilution (an increase in the fluid content of the blood) occurs. Therefore, anemia may occur if diet is not supplemented with iron.

Systolic blood pressure remains relatively constant during rest (contractile phase of the cardiac cycle). In contrast, diastolic blood pressure (relaxation phase of the cardiac cycle) decreases until mid-pregnancy, then increases to normal levels by delivery. Possibly, as blood volume increases, a decrease in peripheral resistance occurs, therefore lowering diastolic blood pressure.

Pulmonary Changes

The rib cage becomes elevated due to the pressure exerted on the diaphragm by the growing uterus. The changes become obvious during the

TABLE 9-1   American College of Obstetricians and Gynecologists Exercise Guidelines for Pregnancy.

Maternal heart rate should not exceed 140 bpm.

Strenuous activities should not exceed 15 minutes duration.

No exercise in the supine position after fourth month gestation.

No exercises employing the valsalva maneuver (holding the breath while exerting force).

Caloric intake adequate for pregnancy and exercise needs.

Maternal core temperature should not exceed 38° C or 101° F.

second trimester and lead to an inspiratory capacity increase (maximum volume of air inspired after an expiration), and a reduction in functional residual capacity (volume in the lungs after expiration at rest). Oxygen consumption (an indirect measurement of energy expenditure) increases approximately 10 to 20 percent above nonpregnant levels. Oxygen consumption increases because of the added workload associated with weight gain. Minute ventilation (the volume of air inspired or expired in one minute) increases approximately 40 percent. This may occur because of the rib cage expansion. Breathing deeply becomes difficult, so to maintain a normal vital capacity (combined volume of air with a maximal inspiration and expiration) minute ventilation must increase. Consequently, hyperventilation (excessive lung ventilation caused by an increased depth and frequency of breathing; usually resulting in an excess elimination of CO^2) frequently occurs throughout pregnancy. Ventilation is increased due to deeper breathing.

Hormonal Changes

Various hormonal changes affect maintenance of body temperature, electrolyte balance, cervical softening and so forth. However, current research is inconclusive concerning exercise effect on hormonal changes. The two main steroidal hormones, estrogen and progesterone, are predominantly produced in the placenta. Progesterone is involved in the maintenance of body temperature and electrolyte balance, and increases substantially 48 hours prior to delivery. Estrogen increases constantly from a nonpregnant level.

The hormone relaxin is produced in the ovaries and may prevent premature labor. Also, the hormone increases cervical softening and may relax tissues surrounding the joints.

Weight Gain

The average maternal weight gain is 26.5 lbs. Approximately 20.25 lbs. are the products of conception: fetus, amniotic fluid, placenta, fluid gain, breast and uterine tissue gain. The remaining 6 lbs. is increased fat and lean body mass.

Effects of Exercise

Information concerning human maternal and fetal response to exercise is limited. However, current research indicates that exercise at moderate intensity levels in apparently healthy pregnant women is beneficial.

Cardiovascular Effects.   The effect of endurance training results in cardiac hypertrophy (enlargement of the cardiac muscle), a slight increased oxygen consumption, increased stroke volume, cardiac output, and total blood volume, and a decreased resting heart rate. The increased blood volume allows for an increased ability for carrying oxygen to the tissues. Thus, with an increased ability to carry oxygen and more blood pumped per beat, the entire cardiovascular system becomes more efficient.

In comparison, pregnancy itself results in cardiac hypertrophy, increased stroke volume, cardiac output, and total blood volume. In contrast to endurance training, resting heart rates increase throughout pregnancy. Therefore, the effect of an endurance training program may be masked by the accompanying changes due to the pregnancy itself.

Temperature Effects.   Aerobic exercise raises core temperature. However, the rise is dependent upon intensity of exercise, humidity, and hydration level. The harder a person exercises, the higher the body core temperature rises. Temperatures in excess of 101° F have been associated with neural tube defects. The neural tube develops into the fetal brain and spinal cord. These defects are relatively rare (2 per 1,000 births) and are also associated with radiation exposure and rubella.

Dehydration Effects.   In addition, dehydration should be avoided during the latter stages of pregnancy, because dehydration may precipitate premature labor. Consequently, pregnant women should avoid high-intensity long duration aerobic activities. Exercise should be avoided in high temperatures and/or high humidity.

In relation to the fetus during exercise, two factors are important: 1) maternal core temperature, and 2) oxygen supply throught the placenta. The fetus is completely dependent upon the mother for nutrient and oxygen supply. The placenta supplies oxygen and nutrients, and is the main mechanism to control fetal temperatures. In addition, waste product removal is controlled by uterine, placental, and ultimately maternal blood flow.

During prenatal exercise, a selective redistribution of blood flow to the working muscles occurs. Consequently, blood flow is reduced to the splanchnic (abdominal and thoracic) organs, possibly reducing uterine and placental blood. Therefore, if the blood supply is limited through the placenta, the fetus may receive a decreased oxygen and nutrient supply. This may result in an increased body temperature and potential fetal distress. However, research is inconclusive in this area. Several studies report that while uterine blood flow decreases, placental blood flow remains within normal levels. This suggests that the fetus may have a protective mechanism for blood flow regulation.

Depending on the extent of blood redistribution, various effects on fetal heart rate may occur. For example, fetal heart rate may be affected by: 1) maternal core temperature, 2) oxygen supply through the placenta, 3) fetal hypoxia (reduction of oxygen to the tissues despite adequate blood flow), 4) fetal movements, and 5) time of day. The consideration is whether maternal exercise compromises fetal heart rate (FHR) through limited oxygen supply.

Fetal HR Effects.   Fetal heart rates below 110 bpm for a minimum of three minutes are considered fetal distress. Normal third trimester FHRs are approximately 120 to 160 beats per minute (bpm) and vary 10 to 25 bpm. Increases and decreases within these limits are considered an important indicator of fetal nervous system development and well-being.

Studies of fetal heart rate response to maternal exercise report inconsistent results. That is, FHR has been found to increase, decrease, or remain stable both during and following exercise. Therefore, conclusions cannot be generalized concerning fetal response. The correlation between fetal bradycardia (reduced heart rate below 100 bpm) and fetal hypoxia has not been determined.

Nutritional Concerns and Effects.   Even though research has examined many physiological changes during pregnancy, few studies have compared maternal weight gain and exercise intensity. The differences in maternal weight gain may exist due to: 1) exercise intensity and duration, 2) caloric intake levels, and 3) conceptus weight (fetus, placenta, amniotic fluid).

During pregnancy the energy demand is approximately 100 to 300 kcal per day above nonpregnant levels, primarily because of an increase in the basal metabolic rate. For sedentary individuals, caloric intake must increase slightly to maintain normal weight gain during pregnancy. However, a greater caloric intake is needed to maintain normal weight gain when exercising during pregnancy.

Current research does not show that human fetal birth weight is affected by maternal exercise. Typically the studies demonstrate similar birth weights between women who exercise and those who do not. It appears that fetal birth weight is more dependent upon adequate nutritional intake.

Recommendations for the Aerobic Dance Participant

All pregnant women participating in regular aerobic exercise should consult with their physicians concerning possible contraindications. The program for each pregnant participant should be individualized for their current needs.

Some pregnant women develop conditions that preclude their participation in an aerobic program (Table 9-2). A medical questionnaire should screen for these conditions. If any of these conditions surface, the pregnant participant should then be disallowed participation.

Many pregnant women develop conditions that limit participation in your program. Pregnant women who suffer from the following conditions should participate only under direct physician approval and supervision (Table 9-3).

The American College of Obstetricians and Gynecologists advises that enrollment in a new aerobic program or increase in intensity of a current program should be avoided. Previously sedentary women should begin exercise with a mild walking program.

Exercise in hot and/or humid climates should be avoided. The participant should be encouraged to drink plenty of fluids before, during, and after exercise. Most women will naturally decrease their aerobic workout intensity as pregnancy progresses. However, a few will attempt their usual high intensities. These women should be encouraged to taper their programs.

Pregnant women should be encouraged to participate in nonweight bearing activities, or at least avoid many of the jarring and bouncing movements associated with aerobic dance. A support bra especially designed for active women should be worn. Aerobic shoes should be a high quality and provide good support. Clothing should be light cotton and should breath easily to avoid excess temperature increase. Support hose will reduce edema in the legs and ankles, and help prevent blood pooling in the legs.

TABLE 9-2   Absolute Contraindications.

Ruptured Membranes

Bleeding from the Vagina

Premature Labor

Multiple Gestation

Heart Disease

Placenta Previa (a placenta that develops in the lower uterine segment)

Incompetent Cervix (a cervix that is abnormally prone to dilate in the second trimester causing premature delivery)

History of Three or More Spontaneous Abortions or Miscarriages

---

TABLE 9-3 Relative Contraindications.

High Blood Pressure (generally above 140/90 for an extended period of time)

Anemia (a deficiency in the oxygen carrying capacity of the blood) or other Blood Disorders

Diabetes

Thyroid Disease

Excessive Obesity (in excess of 35 percent body fat)

Extreme Underweight (13 percent or less body fat)

History of Precipitous Labor (an undue rapid labor)

Palpitations (irregular rapid heart beat) or Irregular Heart Rhythms

History of Intrauterine Growth Retardation (subnormal fetal growth in the uterus)

Breech Presentation in the Last Trimester (delivery of the fetus with the feet or buttocks appearing first)

History of Bleeding During Present Pregnancy

Extreme Sedentary Lifestyle

Women should wear minipads if urinary incontinence occurs. This problem is common as the fetus places increased pressure on the bladder.

Implications for the Aerobic Dance Instructor

As an instructor, potential problems can be avoided through designing exercises that have the following components:

1. Provide an adequate warm-up, because of the possible increased joint laxity during pregnancy.
2. Encourage gentle, longer duration stretching.
3. Avoid movements that place the joints in extreme hyperflexion or hyperextension, especially the knee and hip regions.
4. Avoid movements in forward and side bending, and cross body movements. Any movement that the growing abdomen will impede should be eliminated, such as touching an elbow to the opposite knee.
5. Activities that require the center of gravity to move out of the line of gravity should be eliminated. Balance is difficult to maintain during exercise, the larger a women's abdomen becomes.
6. Utilize low-impact aerobics rather than the high-impact movements.
7. Avoid abrupt changes in direction, fast movements, and quick turns.
8. Limit high intensity aerobic exercise to approximately 15 minutes, and concentrate on form and control.
9. Eliminate any exercise involving the valsalva maneuver.
10. Encourage controlled breathing during all phases of the exercise session.
11. Finally, provide and encourage an adequate cool-down and rest period to avoid pooling of the blood in the lower extremities, dizziness, and hyperthermia (excessive heat increase).

Many of these problems require immediate medical attention and help should be summoned. If pregnant women should suffer from any of the following they should immediately stop exercise and consult with their physicians: 1) fainting, 2) feeling of disorientation, 3) extreme nausea, 4) sharp pains in the chest or abdomen, 5) vaginal bleeding, 6) loss of fluid from the vagina, 7) blurred vision, 8) severe or continuous headaches, 9) extreme temperature changes, or marked swelling or fluid retention.

A Final Note

Most women who have exercised previously can safely participate during pregnancy. The role of the instructor is to monitor and design activities that are safe and enjoyable for all participants. The pregnant woman presents physiological and mechanical concerns that may be best addressed in a specific prenatal aerobic exercise class. While intermingling in a regular exercise class is beneficial socially and emotionally, the program may not adequately administer to the specific needs of the pregnant women. Regular aerobic exercise should help pregnant women feel better physically and emotionally, improve posture, increase energy levels, reduce stress levels, and possibly reduce excess weight gain.

A Final Note About Aerobic Dance Instruction

We have discussed the five values that we deem important to become an adequate and effective aerobic dance instructor. We fervently believe that to be successful and to feel fulfilled, an instructor must be:

1. Committed to Fitness
2. Educated about Exercise Science
3. Skilled as a Teacher
4. Competent and Able to Apply the Knowledge and Skill, and
5. Certified by a Reputable Agency

Teaching aerobic dance can be challenging and exciting; it depends on your perspective and dedication to knowledge. The rewards from teaching aerobic dance are the same as teaching any sport, activity, or subject: love, enjoyment, and fulfillment. May you experience the joy we have in aerobic dance instruction.

References

AMERICAN ACADEMY OF ORTHOPEDIC SURGEONS. (1984). *Athletic training and sports medicine*. Chicago: American Academy of Orthopedic Surgeons.

AMERICAN COLLEGE OF OBSTETRICIANS AND GYNECOLOGISTS. (1985). *Exercise during pregnancy and the postnatal period*. Washington, D.C., Author.

AMERICAN HEART ASSOCIATION. (1984). Report of Inter-Society Commission for Heart Disease Resources. *Circulation, 70*, 157A-205A.

AMERICAN HEART ASSOCIATION. (1986). *Heart facts*. Dallas, TX: Author.

ARMSTRONG, R.B. (1984). Mechanisms of exercise-induced delayed onset muscular soreness: A brief review. *Medicine and Science in Sports and Exercise, 16*, 529–538.

ARNHEIM, D. D. (1985). *Modern principles of athletic training*. St. Louis: Times Mirror/Mosby Publ. Co.

ARTAL, R., & WISWELL, R. A. (1985). *Exercise in Pregnancy*. Baltimore: Williams and Wilkens.

ASTRAND, P., & RODAHL, K. (1977). *Textbook of Work Physiology*. New York: McGraw Hill Book Co.

BRAY, G.A. (1979). Obesity in America. *International Journal of Obesity, 3*, 363–375.

BROOKS, G. A., & FAHEY, T. D. (1984). *Exercise Physiology: Human Bioenergetics and its Applications*. New York: John Wiley & Sons.

COOPER, P. G. (1987). *Aerobics theory & practice*. Costa Mesa: HDL Communications.

COOPER, K. H. (1982). *The aerobics program for total well-being*. New York: Bantam Books.

COOPER, K. H., POLLOCK, M. L., MARTIN, R. P., WHITE, S. R., LINNERRUD, A.C., & JACKSON, A. (1976). Physical fitness levels vs. selected coronary risk factors: A cross-sectional study. *Journal of the American Medical Association, 236*, 166–169.

DALE, E., MULLINAX, K. M., BRYAN, D. H., & WOODRUFF, N. H. (1982). Exercise during pregnancy: effects on the fetus. *Canadian Journal of Applied Sport Sciences, 7*, 98–103.

DeLORME, T. L., & WATKINS, A. L. (1948). Techniques of progressive resistance exercise. *Archives of Physical Medicine, 29*, 263–273.

DEVRIES, H. A. (1980). *Physiology of exercise for physical education and athletics.* (3rd ed.). Dubuque, IA: Wm C. Brown.

DRESSENDORFER, R. H., & GOODLIN, R. C. (1980). Fetal heart rate response to maternal exercise testing. *The Physician and Sportsmedicine, 8,* 91–94.

FAHEY, T. (1979). *What to do about athletic injuries.* New York: Butterick.

FOOD AND NUTRITION BOARD. (1980). *Recommended dietary allowances, ninth revised edition.* Washington, DC: National Research Council of the National Academy of Sciences.

FOX, E. L., & MATHEWS, D. K. (1981). *The Physiological Basis of Physical Education and Athletics* (3rd ed.). Philadelphia: Saunders College Publishing.

GAUTHIER, M. M. (1986). Guidelines for exercise during pregnancy: too little or too much? *The Physician and Sportsmedicine, 14,* 162–169.

GELDER, N. V. (1987). *Aerobic dance-exercise instructor manual.* San Diego: International Dance-Exercise Association Foundation.

GETCHELL, L. (1979). *Physical fitness: A way of life.* (2nd ed.). New York: John Wiley & Sons.

GIBBONS, L. W., BLAIR, S. N., COOPER, K. H., & SMITH, M. (1983). Association between coronary heart disease risk factors and physical fitness in healthy adult women. *Circulation, 67,* 977–983.

GIRDANO, D. A., DUSEK, D., & EVERLY, G. S. (1985). *Experiencing health.* Englewood Cliffs, NJ: Prentice Hall.

GORSKI, J. (1985). Exercise during pregnancy: maternal and fetal responses. A brief overview. *Medicine and Science in Sports and Exercise, 17,* 407–416.

HARRIS, LOUIS AND ASSOCIATES, INC. (1979). *The Perrier Study: Fitness in America.* New York: Author.

HESSON, J. L. (1985). *Weight training for life.* Englewood, NJ: Morton Pub. Co.

HYTTEN, F., & CHAMBERLAIN, G. (1980). *Clinical Physiology in Obstetrics.* St. Louis: Blackwell Scientific Publications.

KATCH, F. I., & MCARDLE. (1983). *Nutrition, weight control, and exercise* (2nd ed.). Philadelphia: Lea & Febiger.

KRAUS, H., & RAAB, W. (1961). *Hypokinetic disease.* Springfield, IL: Charles C. Thomas.

KREIGHBAUM, E., & BARTHELS, K. M. (1985). *Biomechanics: a qualitative approach for studying human movement* (2nd ed.). Minneapolis: Burgess Pub. Co.

METROPOLITAN LIFE INSURANCE COMPANY. (1959). New weight standards for men and women. *Statistical Bulletin Metropolitan Life Insurance Company, 40,* 1–4.

METROPOLITAN LIFE INSURANCE COMPANY. (1983). *1983 Metropolitan height and weight tables.* New York: Author.

NIEMAN, D. C. (1986). *The Sports Medicine Fitness Course.* Palo Alto: Bull Publishing Company.

PRESIDENT'S COUNCIL ON PHYSICAL FITNESS AND SPORTS. (1972). *National Adult Physical Fitness Survey.* Princeton, N.J.: Opinion Research Corporation.

SAGE, G. H. (1977). *Introduction to motor behavior: a neuropsychological approach* (2nd ed.). Reading: Addison-Wesley Pub. Co.

SAGE, G. H. (1984). *Motor learning and control: a neuropsychological approach.* Dubuque: Wm C. Brown Pub.

SHARKEY, B. J. (1984). *Physiology of fitness* (2nd ed.). Champaign, IL: Human Kinetics Publishers.

STOLL, S. K. (1986). *The University fitness aerobic, lifting, diet, and nutrition program.* Moscow: University of Idaho Press.

TAFARI, N., NAEYE, R. L., & GOBEZIE, A. (1980). Effects of maternal undernutrition and heavy physical work during pregnancy on birth weight. *British Journal of Obstetrics and Gynecology, 89,* 222–226.

TORG, J. S. (1982). Athletic footwear and orthopedic appliances. In J. S. Torg (ed.), *Clinics in sports medicine* (pp. 157–175). Philadelphia: W. B. Saunders Co.

TORTORA G. J., & ANAGNOSTAKOS, N. P. (1978). *Principles of Anatomy and Physiology* (2nd ed.). New York: Canfield Press.

WILMORE, J. H. (1986). *Sensible fitness.* Champaign, IL: Leisure Press.

Index

A

Abdominals, curl-up, 27–30
Acoustics, aerobic dance program, 97–98
Aerobic conditioning effects:
  on aging,16
  on arthritis, 15–16
  on arthritis, 15–16
  fat to body mass, 14
  lipoproteins, changes in, 13–14
  on lower back pain, 15
  lowered blood pressure, 13
  metabolic rate increase, 14–15
Aerobic dance, defintion of, 5
Aerobic dance programs:
  acoustic, 97-98
  aerboic dance session, 94
  consent form, 89, 90
  cool-down, 93, 94
  dress for, 99–100
  equipment, 99
  facilities, 92–94
  muscular stength building, 91–94
  pre-exercise evaluation form, 88–89
  pre-exercise scrccning, 87–88
  shoes, 100–101
  showers, 98
  sound system, 98
  ventilation, 96–97
  warm-up, 89, 91
Age:
  and aerobic conditioning, 16
  and injuries, 155
  and type of aerboic class, 104
Amenorrhea, athletic, 56
Anaerobic system, 21
Ankle weights, 99, 153
Anorexia nervosa, 56–57
Arthritis, and aerobic conditioning, 15–16

B

Back:
  dorsal-curl, 35
  flexibility exercise, 47–48
Back pain, lower, and aerobic
  conditioning, 15
Bend and stethe, movements for, 127
Bicycle ergometers, 17
Blood pooling, 93